FUNDAMENTALS

Fundamentals of

Care

A Textbook for Health and Social Care Assistants

FUNDAMENTALS

Fundamentals of

Care

A Textbook for Health and Social Care Assistants

IAN PEATE OBE

Professor of Nursing, Head of School
School of Health Studies, Gibraltar
Visiting Professor
St George's, University of London; Kingston University, London

WILEY Blackwell

Library of Congress Cataloging-in-Publication data are available

ISBN: 9781119212201

A catalogue record for this book is available from the British Library.

Wiley also publishes its books in a variety of electronic formats. Some content that appears in print may not be available in electronic books.

Cover image: © Dean Mitchell/Getty Images.

Chapter opener images reproduced courtesy of Anthony Peate.

Set in 10/12pt Myriad by SPi Global, Pondicherry, India.
Printed and bound in Singapore by Markono Print Media Pte Ltd.

1   2017

Contents

vii

Contents

Preface

The provision of health and social care along with support provided to people is changing and will continue to change. In the healthcare sector in England there is to be a new nursing associate role, to provide greater support for nurses and help to bridge the gap between healthcare support workers and nurses. The nursing associate will be trained through the apprenticeship route. Once trained they will work alongside healthcare support workers to deliver hands-on care, freeing up time for existing nurses so they can use their specialist training to focus on clinical duties and take more of a lead in decisions around patient care.

This text has been written for staff who are new in their role as well as for those who are already employed as a healthcare assistant, assistant practitioner, care support worker or those who provide support where there is direct contact with people receiving services. The book will also be suitable for those who are contemplating undertaking the role of nursing associate. Adult social care workers who provide direct care in residential and nursing homes or a hospice, or home care workers will also find the content of this book applicable to their sphere of work. It is acknowledged that roles undertaken will vary in different health and social care settings.

In England in April 2015, the Care Certificate was introduced. The Government now expects that all those working as healthcare assistants and adult social care workers will undertake learning related to the standards of the Care Certificate as part of their induction programme. The Cavendish Review, published in July 2013, was one of the key drivers for the creation of the Care Certificate.

An Independent Review into Healthcare Assistants and Support Workers in the NHS and social care settings was undertaken in 2013 (Cavendish, 2013). It was estimated that there are over 1.3 million frontline staff who are not registered with a regulatory authority but who now deliver most of hands-on care in hospitals, care homes and the homes of individuals (Cavendish, 2013). The Cavendish Review (requested by the Secretary of State for Health in the wake of the publication of the Francis Inquiry into Mid-Staffordshire NHS Foundation Trust) examined what could be done to ensure that unregistered staff in the NHS and social care treat all people with care and compassion.

The review revealed how disconnected the systems are that care for the public, and amongst other things proposed new common training standards across health and social care, grounded in what the best employers already do. It proposed a Certificate of Fundamental Care, written in plain English, to make a positive statement about caring necessitating the Care Quality Commission (CQC) to require all workers to have achieved this Certificate prior to working unsupervised.

There are often inconsistent approaches to the training and development of healthcare assistants and adult social care workers, with varying quality. The Care Certificate has been created to address these variances. The Care Certificate consists of 15 standards; these standards address the Code of Conduct for Healthcare Support Workers and Adult Social Care Workers in England but can also be applied to the three other UK countries.

The Care Certificate applies across the health and social care sectors and is portable between sectors and organisations. The Care Certificate covers the learning outcomes, competencies and standards of behaviour that are expected of support workers in the health and social care sectors.

The Care Certificate defines the required values, behaviours and competencies that carers must demonstrate, aiming to ensure that the care and support offered is caring, compassionate and of a high quality.

Each of the standards related to the Care Certificate has specific outcomes and competencies that are associated with them; these must be achieved in order for one to be eligible for a Care Certificate; assessment of both knowledge and competence is required. It is not the purpose of this book to replace the Care Certificate standards; however, working through the various chapters will enable the reader to develop their knowledge and apply this to their work.

The Care Certificate cannot be completed through completion of e-learning or completing a workbook alone. E-learning or workbooks can support the attainment of knowledge but the assessment of the required skills has to be undertaken in the workplace.

The chapters

There are 18 chapters in the book. The first chapter provides an overview of health and social care provision, and Chapter 2 outlines the importance of working with others as a member of a team. Fifteen chapters are dedicated to the Care Certificate, and the final chapter, Chapter 18, provides support to the health and social care worker in addressing questions, queries and concerns that they may have or have experienced in the workplace.

The text adopts an engaging practical approach, and where appropriate practice exercises have been incorporated encouraging the reader to stop, look, listen and act, to take stock and carry out activities pertinent to the chapter. Where appropriate the student will be encouraged to interact with chapter content by completing activities, engendering curiosity. Reflection comes in the form of thinking activities.

Where appropriate at the beginning of the chapter the outcomes associated with each standard will be reproduced, contextualising and focusing the reader on the chapter content and relevance to the Care Certificate. There is an opportunity for readers to self-assess. Readers can rate their current knowledge and skills prior to reading each chapter in relation to the chapter content. Each chapter ends with a case study reflecting chapter content. A resource file is included, inside which are resources that will help the reader to seek support and access further information should this be needed. These include links to the World Wide Web or references to appropriate literature.

An annotated bibliography has been provided. The purpose is to provide the reader with further information to support their learning.

What's in a name?

The terms used to describe the relationship between those who provide care and offer support and those who are the recipients of those services vary; for example, user, service user, consumer, patient, client, survivor and expert are used. This text uses the terms 'people' or 'person' to describe those who receive or access services.

Terminology, job titles and roles in healthcare also vary; these can include: Assistant Practitioner, Care Assistant, Healthcare Support Worker, Maternity Support Worker, Nursing Assistant, Occupational Therapy Assistant, Physiotherapy Assistant, Radiography Assistant, Speech and Language Therapy Assistant and Senior Care Assistant. In Adult Social Care these roles and titles may include: Activities Worker, Day Care Assistant, Day Care Officer, Domiciliary Care Worker, Home Care Worker, Nursing Home or Hospice Nursing Assistant, Personal Assistant, Reablement Assistant, Residential Care Worker, Senior Home Care Worker and Support Worker.

I have enjoyed writing this text and I sincerely hope that you enjoy reading it and that you are able to apply the content to the care and support that you offer people.

Ian Peate
Gibraltar

Reference

Cavendish, C. (2013) The Cavendish Review. An Independent Review into Healthcare Assistants and Support Workers in the NHS and Social Care Settings. Available at: https://www.gov.uk/government/uploads/system/uploads/attachment_data/file/236212/Cavendish_Review.pdf (accessed August 2016).

Acknowledgements

I would like to thank the library staff at Gibraltar Health Authority for their help. My partner, Jussi Lahtinen, for his encouragement, and Mrs Frances Cohen who, without hesitation, provides me with support and inspiration.

How to use your textbook

Features contained within your textbook

Care certificate outcomes lists the key learning points from the chapter.

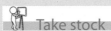

Care certificate outcomes

1. Understand your own role.
2. Work in ways that have been agreed with your employer.
3. Understand working relationships in health and social care.
4. Work in partnership with others.

Take stock allows you to rate your current knowledge and skills prior to reading the chapter.

Take stock

Rate your current knowledge and skills prior to reading this chapter. Put a tick in the box that you think applies to you with regards to the standard being discussed:

'Thinking cap' boxes give further insight into conditions and cases.

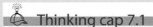

Thinking cap 7.1

Respect

Can you think of a time (at work or in a social setting) when you have felt disrespect? What made you feel like this? Did you do anything about this? If so what and if not why not?

'Stop, look, respond' boxes provide exercises to encourage you to think what you might do in a certain situation.

 Stop, look, respond 8.1

Types of communication

Write notes and if possible give examples of where and when you have used the types of communication below.

Case scenarios give a real-life case based around the chapter content.

 Case scenario 3.1

Folami

Folami works as an activities worker in a dementia care centre. Folami is assisting the occupational therapist (Jay), and Jay and Folami have worked together for a number of years. The occupational therapist has set up a range of activities for a group of six people he is working with. The aim of the session is to enhance function, promote relationships and social participation, and to find ways for those members of the group to enjoy life. One member of the group, Marie, becomes disorientated and tends to wander; preserving Marie's safety is a key issue.

Resource file lists some places you can look for more information.

 Resource file

British Institute of Human Rights
An organisation providing people with authoritative and accessible information regarding human rights.
https://www.bihr.org.uk

Stonewall
A lesbian, gay, bisexual and transgender rights charity.
http://www.stonewall.org.uk

The Equality Trust
The Equality Trust works to improve the quality of life in the UK by reducing economic inequality.
https://www.equalitytrust.org.uk/resources

Chapter 1

Health and social care provision in the UK

Care certificate outcomes

There are no care certificate outcomes for this chapter. This chapter aims to:

- Introduce the reader to health and care provision across the UK.
- Emphasise the fact that the four different countries of the UK adopt different approaches to care provision whilst still being a part of the wider National Health Service.
- Offer the reader some insight into past and present issues surrounding health and social care.

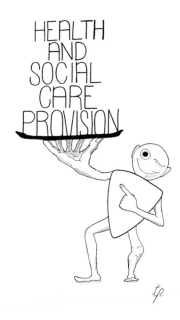

Fundamentals of Care: A Textbook for Health and Social Care Assistants, First Edition. Ian Peate.
© 2017 John Wiley & Sons Ltd. Published 2017 by John Wiley & Sons Ltd.

Take stock

Rate your current knowledge and skills prior to reading this chapter. Put a tick in the box that you think applies to you with regards to the standard being discussed.

Key:
I know this I have a good level of knowledge or skills regarding this aspect of the standard. I make use of the knowledge and skills identified on a regular basis, feeling confident in my ability and performance. I do not need a refresher.
Satisfactory My level of knowledge and standard of skills meet the criteria associated with the standard. I use the skills and knowledge from time to time. I might not always feel confident in my capability, I would benefit from a refresher.
I require a review I do not feel that I have the skills and/or the knowledge that would enable me to meet the standard in a confident and competent way. The knowledge and skills I used to have are no longer valid. I will require a refresher.
This is new to me I have never worked in a caring role before or I have never covered this topic before. I will need further training and development in this area.

Standard	Self-assessment			
Understand health and social care provision in the UK	☐ I know this	☐ Satisfactory	☐ I should review this	☐ This is new to me
Discuss the role and function of the NHS nationally and locally	☐ I know this	☐ Satisfactory	☐ I should review this	☐ This is new to me
Describe how health and social care services are regulated and monitored	☐ I know this	☐ Satisfactory	☐ I should review this	☐ This is new to me
Highlight aspects of health and social care offered and provided by the NHS, the private and voluntary sectors	☐ I know this	☐ Satisfactory	☐ I should review this	☐ This is new to me
Differentiate between primary, secondary and tertiary services	☐ I know this	☐ Satisfactory	☐ I should review this	☐ This is new to me
Develop an insight into the assessment of health and social care needs for individuals and communities	☐ I know this	☐ Satisfactory	☐ I should review this	☐ This is new to me

Introduction

The ways in which health and social care provision are provided have changed over the years and it is very likely that they will continue to change. The four countries of the United Kingdom (UK) – Northern Ireland, Wales, England and Scotland – each have devolved responsibilities for the provision of health and social care service within their borders. This means that each country sets its own priorities for care provision. Often, because of these transferred responsibilities (transferred from central government), discussing the issue in a general manner can become complex. The focus of this chapter will be predominantly on the provision of health and social care service in England.

An historical view

Care, being cared for, providing care is an essential human need in order for the full development, maintenance and sustaining of human beings. The tradition of caring has often been associated with women – a female activity that focuses on the individual, the family and groups of people. Care and cure are two very different entities and it could be implied that throughout history care has not been awarded the same importance as cure. Cure it could be suggested has gained more attention because of the public recognition of a range of supposedly lifesaving and life-sustaining new technologies and, tentatively, because it is very often associated with males, whereas care is seen as a traditional female activity. However, there cannot be any curing without caring, and the notion of care has been rooted in our history through examples such as religious (or spiritual), social, political, educational and economic contexts.

Health and disease are ever-present factors of the human state, and throughout history the need for some kind of support and care of individuals and populations has varied. People have always helped other people during times of need (there is also evidence where people have failed to respond to the needs of others), paving the way for the development of systems of care and the fundamental beginnings of health and social care as we know it today. We are all likely to be recipients of care.

The National Health Service

On 5 July 1948, the National Health Service (NHS) was established with the aim of healthcare being free at the point of delivery. Figure 1.1 provides a timeline concerning the NHS since its inception in 1948.

The NHS in the four countries

There are several differences between NHS services in England and the other three home countries:

- Northern Ireland has a fully integrated health and social care service and Scotland has passed legislation to achieve this goal.
- Scotland and Wales have integrated boards (as opposed to trusts) that commission services at a local level.
- Scotland has the Scottish Intercollegiate Guidelines Network (SIGN) for their clinical guidance as opposed to the National Institute for Health and Care Excellence (NICE).

Scotland

In Scotland health and social care policy and funding are the responsibility of the Health and Social Care Directorates of the Scottish Government. There are over 160,000 staff who work across 14 regional NHS Boards, seven Special NHS Boards and one public health body. Around 12,000 of these healthcare staff are engaged under independent contractor arrangements.

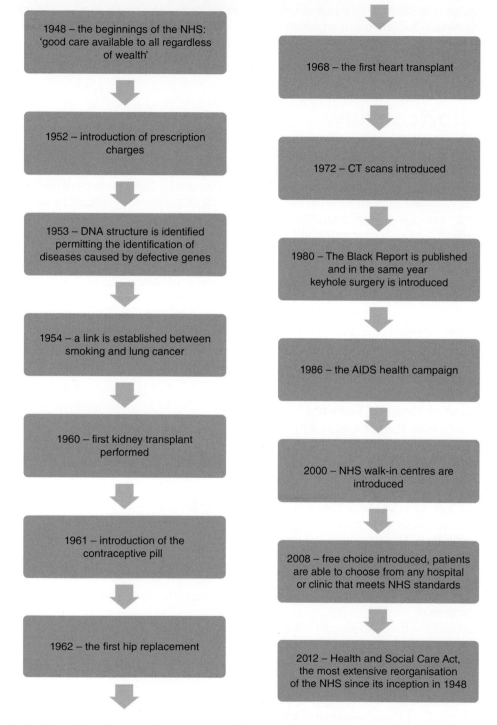

Figure 1.1 Some key dates and events since the inception of the NHS. *Source*: http://www.nhs.uk/ Tools/Pages/NHSTimeline.aspx

The NHS in Scotland is completely devolved and responsibility for it lies wholly with the Scottish Government. The Cabinet Secretary for Health and Wellbeing and Scottish Government set out their national objectives and priorities for the NHS that should be delivered and monitored via NHS Boards and Special NHS Boards.

In 2004 the 14 NHS Boards were replaced by trusts, which cover all of Scotland. These are all-purpose organisations that plan, commission and deliver NHS services for their respective area. They take overall responsibility for the health of their communities and commission all services including GP, dental, community care and hospital care. These boards are also required to work together on a regional and national basis ensuring that specialist healthcare – such as neurosurgery – is commissioned in an effective manner. Locally the boards have representation or partnerships with community health and social care teams, and there is also a close involvement of local authorities, patients and the public.

The population of Scotland is estimated to be in the region of 5.3 million, with a healthcare budget of around £13 billion.

Northern Ireland

The healthcare service in Northern Ireland offers health and social care to its population and is administered by the Department of Health, Social Services and Public Safety.

The Health and Social Care Board carries overall responsibility for the commissioning of services and it does this through five Local Commissioning Groups. The five Local Commissioning Groups have a responsibility for commissioning health and social care and do this by addressing the needs of their local population.

There are five Health and Social Care Trusts that have responsibility for providing an integrated health and social care service in their regions. The Northern Ireland Ambulance Service is seen as a sixth trust.

There is a Patient and Client Council that exists to provide an independent voice for patients, carers and communities. An independent organisation, the Regulation and Quality Improvement Authority, encourages continuous improvement through a programme of inspections.

The Public Health Agency is charged with the responsibility to improve health and wellbeing, provide health protection and input directly into commissioning, and does this through the Health and Social Care Board.

The population of Northern Ireland is estimated to be in the region of 1.8 million, with a healthcare budget of around £4.3 billion.

Wales

In Wales the NHS is devolved, and the Welsh Government assumes responsibility. There are seven Local Health Boards that plan, secure and deliver healthcare services for their populations.

There are three national trusts in Wales:

1. The Welsh Ambulance Services
2. Velindre NHS Trust (providing specialist services in cancer and other national support)
3. A Public Health body for Wales

Representing the health and wellbeing interests of the public in their districts are seven Community Health Councils (CHCs). The Board of Community Health Councils in Wales is responsible for monitoring the performance of the CHCs, the conduct of members and performance of officers as well as operating a Complaints Procedure. It is the aim of the CHC to make sure that when people across Wales speak about their NHS, those responsible for providing health services listen – and act.

The population of Wales is estimated to be in the region of 3.2 million, with a healthcare budget of around £6.5 billion.

England

High-quality care for all, now and for future generations, is the mission of NHS England. NHS England aims to provide everyone with greater control of their health and wellbeing, supporting them to live longer, and enjoy healthier lives by providing high-quality health and care that is compassionate, inclusive and constantly improving. People are said to be at the heart of everything that the NHS does.

The values that underpin the role and function of the NHS are enshrined in the NHS Constitution (Table 1.1).

Stop, look, respond 1.1

The NHS Constitution

In the list below (the values that underpin the NHS) make notes about how, on a daily basis, you make responses to these vales as you offer care to people.

Value	Example
Respect and dignity	
Commitment to the quality of care	
Compassion	
Improving lives	
Working together for patients	

The population of England is estimated to be in the region of 50 million, with a healthcare budget of around £100 billion. The Department of Health (DH) in England provides strategic leadership for public health, the NHS and social care. It is the Secretary of State who has overall responsibility for the work of the DH.

Thinking cap 1.1

Health and social care services

Think about the health and social services in the country where you are working. Compare some of the services that are offered in the other three countries. What are the good things about health and social care services where you work and what could be improved? Do you think any ideas for improvement in services could come from one or more of the other three countries?

Table 1.1 NHS values and the NHS constitution

- Respect and dignity
- Commitment to the quality of care
- Compassion
- Improving lives
- Working together for patients

Provision of services

Various aspects of care are offered and provided by the NHS. However, it must be remembered that it is not just the NHS that provides care; the independent and voluntary sectors also provide care and services to people. The provision of care can take place anywhere where there are people, within the NHS, the private and independent care sector, or in the voluntary care sector. The Health and Social Care Act 2012 provides for fair competition for NHS funding to independent, charity and third-sector healthcare providers; this was introduced with the intention of providing greater choice and control to patients in choosing their care.

The provision of care will be influenced by a number of factors, for example, an ageing population, changing disease patterns, the issue of consumerism and technological advances. Often the provision of care is split between two areas of care:

- acute care;
- chronic care.

The provision of care also takes place within the following settings:

- primary care;
- secondary care;
- tertiary care.

Regulation and monitoring of services

Monitor

To protect the interests of patients in England, Monitor was established as the sector regulator for health services; it is the financial regulator of Foundation Trusts. Monitor issues licences to NHS-funded providers, has responsibility for national pricing (in conjunction with NHS England) and helps commissioners make sure that local services continue if a provider is unable to carry on providing services.

Care Quality Commission

The independent regulator for quality in health and social care in England (including private providers) is the Care Quality Commission (CQC). It registers and inspects:

- hospitals;
- care homes;
- GP surgeries;
- dental practices;
- other healthcare services.

If services are failing to meet fundamental standards of quality and safety, the CQC has the power to:

- issue warnings;
- restrict the service;
- issue a fixed penalty notice;
- suspend or cancel registration;
- prosecute the provider.

Healthwatch

Healthwatch was set up as an independent consumer champion for health and social care. Its function is to represent the public's view on healthcare by gathering views on health and social care locally and nationally. In England every local authority has a Healthwatch. It is anticipated that through the Healthwatch network the voices of those who use the NHS will be heard. Healthwatch gathers these views by undertaking research in local areas, identifying gaps in service provision and feeding into local health commissioning plans.

Professional regulation

The various health and social care professions are regulated by specific regulators (Table 1.2).

Table 1.2   UK professional regulators

Regulator	Profession(s)
General Medical Council (GMC)	The independent regulator of approximately 260,000 doctors in the UK; established to: • Set the standards required of those doctors practising in the UK • Determine which doctors are qualified to work in the UK, oversees their education and training • Ensures doctors continue to meet the standards throughout their careers through a five-yearly cycle of revalidation
Nursing and Midwifery Council (NMC)	The NMC regulates over 670,000 nurses and midwives in the UK. Key responsibilities include: • Setting professional standards of education, training, performance and conduct, and ensuring that these standards are upheld • Investigating nurses and midwives who are thought to fall short of its standards • The ability to take action when a nurse may be putting the safety of patients and others at risk
The General Dental Council (GDC)	The GDC regulates all dental professionals including dentists, dental nurses, technicians and hygienists
The Health and Care Professions Council (HCPC)	Regulates a number of professions including art therapists, biomedical scientists, chiropodists and podiatrists, clinical scientists, dieticians, hearing aid dispensers, occupational therapists, paramedics, social workers in England, and speech and language therapists
The General Pharmaceutical Council (GPhC)	The independent regulator for more than 70,000 pharmacists, technicians and pharmacy premises in the UK. In Northern Ireland this is the Pharmaceutical Society of Northern Ireland
The General Optical Council (GOC)	Regulates approximately 26,000 optometrists, dispensing opticians, student opticians and optical businesses

Table 1.3 Some professionals who deliver primary care

- Social workers
- Teams of nurses
- Prosthetists
- Groups of doctors
- Chiropodists
- Midwives
- Health visitors
- Dentists
- Pharmacists
- Optometrists
- Occupational therapists
- Physiotherapists
- Paramedics
- Speech and language therapists

Primary care services

Most care provision is carried out in the primary care sector; over 95 per cent of care is delivered here. Care is delivered outside hospitals by a range of practitioners (Table 1.3).

Stop, look, respond 1.2

Professional regulation

Match the professionals group listed in Table 1.3 to the regulator below

Regulator	Profession(s)
General Medical Council (GMC)	
Nursing and Midwifery Council (NMC)	
The General Dental Council (GDC)	
The Health and Care Professions Council (HCPC)	
The General Pharmaceutical Council (GPhC)	
The General Optical Council (GOC)	

For many patients, the professional healthcare they require will be provided in the community setting. In some situations, the care provided by and in the primary care sector may not be appropriate, or be unable to meet the needs of the patient. Referral to other services may therefore be required – those services are offered by the secondary care sector.

Secondary care services

This aspect of care provision occurs mainly through the acute hospital setting. The staff who work in this area have more readily available access to specialist and elaborate diagnostic aids and facilities, for example:

- X-ray department;
- magnetic resonance imaging (MRI);
- computed axial tomography (CAT) scans;
- operating theatres;
- special care baby units (SCBU);
- microbiological laboratories;
- various mental health care facilities.

Those who provide care in the primary care setting, for example the social worker, community nurse and GP, could be seen as the 'gatekeepers' to care provision in the secondary care sector, as they may make the necessary referrals to other health and social care providers. The transition from primary care to secondary care should be a seamless move just as the integration of health and social care services should also be seen as a seamless activity. The distinction between primary care and secondary and social care and healthcare are becoming more blurred.

Tertiary care services

Tertiary care is usually available in some larger hospitals. Tertiary care is provided by those with specialist expertise, with available equipment and facilities for caring for the patient with complex healthcare needs, for example:

- intensive care units;
- burns units;
- oncology centres.

It is important to remember that most people receive their care and have their needs met in the primary care setting. Only a few will require secondary services, and even fewer will have to make use of tertiary care services. Health and social care workers and those who support them can be found working in all of these care settings.

Ambulance trusts

These trusts manage emergency care for life-threatening and non-life-threatening illnesses, including the NHS 999 service. In some areas the ambulance trusts have been commissioned to provide non-emergency hospital transport services and/or the NHS 111 service.

 Thinking cap 1.2

NHS 111

What is the NHS 111 service? How does this differ from the 999 service? In what situations might you decide to use the 111 service or the 999 service?

Mental health trusts

Mental health trusts provide community, inpatient and social care services for a wide range of psychiatric and psychological illnesses. Mental health trusts are commissioned and funded by Clinical Commissioning Groups. Mental health services can also be provided by other NHS organisations, the voluntary sector and the private sector.

 ## Stop, look, respond 1.3

Mental health service provision

Mental health services can be provided by a number of organisations other than the NHS, for example, by the voluntary sector and the private sector.

Make a list of who these organisations are and identify if they are from the voluntary sector or the private sector and what their organisation does.

Organisation	Private or voluntary	Role of the organisation

Community health services

These services are delivered by foundation and non-foundation community health trusts. Services include:

- district nurses;
- health visitors;
- school nursing;
- community specialist services;
- hospital at home;
- NHS walk-in centres;
- home-based rehabilitation.

Social care and support

Social care is provided to people who may be having difficulty in managing daily tasks at home and who may need extra support and care. The care and support system can be very complex and confusing, with a number of organisations involved in assessment, arrangement and provision of care. This complexity and confusion can aggravate a person's ability to cope and manage.

Stop, look, respond 1.4

Community health services

Choose one of the community health services above and discuss the role and function of the service. Complete the table.

Chosen service:	
Who works in this service?	
Where is the service located?	
How do people access the service?	
Are service users involved in the development of the service?	
Is this a statutory, private or voluntary service?	

There are several rules and regulations that govern how people pay for care and support or what their entitlements to care and support might be; this too can be difficult to understand. Help and advice is available from the government and also from those in the voluntary and independent sectors, for example the charity Age UK.

Examples of services that are available to help people with care and support needs can include:

- Help at home with shopping, laundry and cleaning.
- Intensive home care including washing, dressing and preparing a meal.
- The provision of 24-hour care in a care home or housing with a care scheme (this is also known as sheltered accommodation).

If a person is in need of care and support, instead of receiving directly funded and arranged services, they can request for cash payments for them to arrange their own care. This approach can provide greater choice and control over how their needs can be best met.

Some people may also be entitled to the provision of equipment and adaptations to help ensure that their home is more suitable in meeting their needs.

Assessment of care needs

There are a number of assessment procedures in place that will establish a person's needs; these are often set by the local authority (eligibility of need). Each local authority has its own assessment procedure.

Each local authority has a duty to assess a person who appears to need care and support. They may need care and support as a result of a serious illness, physical disability, learning disability, mental health problem or frailty because of old age.

This may mean that an assessment is offered even if the person has not specifically requested one. The person can contact their local social services department and request for them to arrange a needs assessment. Usually, an assessment is carried out prior to a service being provided by the social services department of a local authority. If care is needed urgently, then the local authority may be able to meet those needs without performing the assessment.

Table 1.4   The care plan

The care plan must set out:
- The needs identified by the assessment
- Whether and to what extent the needs meet the eligibility criteria
- The needs that the authority is going to meet, and how it intends to do this
- For a person needing care, for which of the desired outcomes care and support could be relevant
- For a carer, the outcomes the carer wishes to achieve and their wishes concerning care provision, work, education and recreation where support could be relevant
- The personal budget
- Information and advice on what can be done to reduce the needs in question and to prevent or delay the development of needs in the future
- Where needs are being met via a direct payment, the needs to be met via the direct payment and the amount and frequency of the payments
- The person's care plan should be individual, and they should be allowed to have as much involvement in the development of the plan as they wish

Reviews of the care plan

The care plan should be reviewed by social services within the first 3 months and then as a minimum at least annually.

Once it has been established by a local authority that a person has needs that conform to the national eligibility criteria, that authority has to ensure that those needs are met. Initially a care and support plan has to be drawn up, or in the case of a carer with eligible needs, a support plan is needed.

A care plan (sometimes this is called a care and support plan, or support plan if the person is a carer) sets out how the person's care and support needs will be met. The person should be fully involved in the preparation of the care plan; they and anyone else they request should also be provided with a written copy (Table 1.4).

If there are eligible needs, the local authority will check that the person normally lives in its area. Social care is not free; it may be that the person will have to contribute towards the cost of meeting their needs. Local authorities will do an assessment to determine if the person will have to contribute and how much this might be.

The local authority should not refuse to meet eligible needs based on cost; however, if there is more than one option, they are allowed to choose what it believes will be the most cost-effective one.

If the person's needs do not meet the national eligibility criteria, the local authority is required to provide information and advice on what support might be available in the community to support the individual.

The person may consider or choose to fund their own care and support in response to the needs that have been identified as a result of the assessment. If the person disagrees with the needs assessment or the care and support plan that has been formulated, there are processes in place that challenge decisions.

Assessment of health needs

Assessing a person's (or population's) health needs requires a systematic approach. The term 'health' is a complex one and can be defined as a positive concept that is associated with social, personal and physical capabilities. It concerns the ability of individuals and their perceptions of their ability to function and to cope with their social and physical environment, as well as with any specific illnesses and with life in general.

Individual healthcare needs are just that, individual; a one-size fits all approach is unacceptable. Needs are identified by the person or in conjunction with healthcare professionals such as a nurse. Assessment tools are used to determine any healthcare deficit.

The needs of populations can be identified by engaging with those populations (including service user groups), and this is done in a number of ways with the aim of listening to and acting on what has been said. A range of health and social care professionals can contribute to identifying needs; these professionals may include clinical health scientists, social workers and doctors.

Chapter summary

- The NHS is there for all of us; it was created out of the ideal that good healthcare should be available to all, irrespective of wealth.
- The provision of health and social care in the UK is complex.
- The four countries of the UK have devolved responsibility for health and social care.
- There are various aspects of care offered and provided by the NHS; the independent and voluntary sectors also provide care and services to people.
- To protect the interests of those who use services, service provision is regulated and monitored.
- Professions are regulated by their professional bodies.
- Care takes place in many places and this includes the primary, secondary and tertiary sectors.
- There are a number of assessment procedures in place that will establish a person's health and social needs.

Case scenario 1.1

Anna

Anna Chosky is a 64-year-old lady who presented to the accident and emergency department accompanied by her daughter (Desirée), who is her main carer. Anna has been experiencing increasingly severe dyspnoea on exertion and progressive oedema of the lower extremities. She reported that her breathlessness and coughing episodes had become particularly severe in the preceding 3 weeks and she was now at the point where she could not stand or walk for more than 1 to 2 minutes without becoming fatigued. Anna had been sleeping on the sofa downstairs. Desirée has been assisting Anna with her personal hygiene needs, doing her shopping, cooking her food and attending to household jobs such as cleaning.

Anna is assessed in the accident and emergency department and is diagnosed with exacerbation of chronic obstructive pulmonary disease (COPD).

She is admitted to a ward and is receiving treatment. After 4 days of treatment she is ready for discharge home and plans are being made with various health and social care agencies, a care plan is being formulated with her. A home visit with the occupational therapist is planned and suitable adjustments to her home environment to provide her with as much independence as possible are being instigated.

In the scenario identify what you think Anna's needs are from a health and social care perspective. How can the health and social services assist Desirée in supporting her mother in her home?

Make notes of any words you do not understand in the scenario and write a definition of these words.

Resource file

Department of Health, Social Services and Public Safety
www.dhsspsni.gov.uk

GIG Cymru NHS Wales
www.wales.nhs.uk

NHS Scotland
www.show.scot.nhs.uk

NHS England
www.england.nhs.uk

Chapter 2

Working with others, teamwork

Care certificate outcomes

There are no care certificate outcomes for this chapter. This chapter aims to:

- Impress on the reader the importance of working together in health and care settings.
- Differentiate between groups and teams.
- Describe teamwork.
- Identify the various team members.
- Appreciate the benefits of effective teamworking for people to whom you offer care and support.
- Know how to be an effective teamworker.

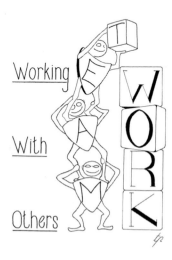

Fundamentals of Care: A Textbook for Health and Social Care Assistants, First Edition. Ian Peate.
© 2017 John Wiley & Sons Ltd. Published 2017 by John Wiley & Sons Ltd.

Take stock

Rate your current knowledge and skills prior to reading this chapter. Put a tick in the box that you think applies to you with regards to the standard being discussed.

Key:
I know this I have a good level of knowledge or skills regarding this aspect of the standard. I make use of the knowledge and skills identified on a regular basis, feeling confident in my ability and performance. I do not need a refresher.
Satisfactory My level of knowledge and standard of skills meet the criteria associated with the standard. I use the skills and knowledge from time to time. I might not always feel confident in my capability. I would benefit from a refresher.
I require a review I do not feel that I have the skills and/or the knowledge that would enable me to meet the standard in a confident and competent way. The knowledge and skills I used to have are no longer valid. I will require a refresher.
This is new to me I have never worked in a caring role before or I have never covered this topic before. I will need further training and development in this area.

Standard	Self-assessment			
Understand the value of working in partnership with others	☐ I know this	☐ Satisfactory	☐ I should review this	☐ This is new to me
Explain the concepts of teams	☐ I know this	☐ Satisfactory	☐ I should review this	☐ This is new to me
Identify team members	☐ I know this	☐ Satisfactory	☐ I should review this	☐ This is new to me
Describe the ways in which teams work	☐ I know this	☐ Satisfactory	☐ I should review this	☐ This is new to me
Identify factors that can enhance teamworking	☐ I know this	☐ Satisfactory	☐ I should review this	☐ This is new to me
Discuss the skills required to be an effective team member	☐ I know this	☐ Satisfactory	☐ I should review this	☐ This is new to me

Introduction

Those who offer care and support to people do not work in isolation; they work with others and also in teams. What is meant and understood by the term 'team' can vary a great deal. In your job you work in partnership with a number of people. Effective teamwork in health and social care delivery can have an immediate and positive impact on safety for all. Working with others requires you to work in partnership in an effective and respectful way. To work effectively you must embrace the concept of effective teamworking. Teamworking, similar to interprofessional working, is defined in many ways and is often used synonymously with group working.

Teamworking

Effective teamworking has the ability to improve cooperation and partnerships and to enhance communications and working practices across various organisational boundaries. Teamworking does not take place in a vacuum; there are many factors that must be taken into consideration, such as the needs and interests of the various stakeholders.

The Health Act 1999 imposes a duty on all NHS organisations to work in partnership. The key aim of some legislation, for instance the Community Care Act 1990, is to promote closer and collaborative partnerships with service users. The aim is to provide those who use services with a service that is seamless and joined up; there is a need for coordination and continuity, and working in and as a team with effective communication channels can help this become a reality.

 ## Stop, look, respond 2.1

Professional groups

Below is a list of different professional groups who you may have to work with in a collaborative manner when providing care or support:

- Physiotherapists
- Dieticians
- Paramedics
- Radiographers
- Occupational therapists
- Speech and language therapists
- Social workers
- Police
- Doctors
- Probation managers
- Audiologists
- Dentists
- Opticians

Each of the above groups has its own unique professional culture. These professional groups have unique professional identities; however, they are expected to come together to work as a professional group, a team.

Now choose three of the professional groups and outline their role and function in relation to the people you care for or offer support to:

1. _____
   _____
   _____
   _____

2. _____
   _____
   _____
   _____

3. _____
   _____
   _____
   _____

The importance of effective teams in health and social care is increasing as a result of a number of factors. For example:

- The increasing complexity of needs.
- An increasingly ageing population.
- An increase in the number of people with chronic disease.
- Technological advances.
- An increase in public expectations.
- The political agenda to ensure health and social provision come closer together.

It is one thing to create a team but another to create teamwork; teams do not work without teamwork. There are many ways to define teamwork; for example, it could be said to be cooperation between those who are working on a task. However, this definition is rather simple. Teamwork exists when a group of people work together in a joined up way towards a common goal, creating a positive working environment, supporting each other to combine individual strengths to improve the team's collective performance. Table 2.1 considers teamworking from a number of perspectives.

 ## Stop, look, respond 2.2

Teams

With regards to Table 2.1, fill in below who you think the various members of the multidisciplinary, interdisciplinary and transdisciplinary teams might be in the place where you work.

Multidisciplinary	Interdisciplinary	Transdisciplinary

In order to provide the best possible care and support that is responsive to a person's individual needs, the health and social care worker has to work in partnership with other professionals, volunteers and carers. These will include paid and unpaid workers as well as friends, family and relatives. Other health professionals will be able to provide you with useful

Table 2.1 Teamworking

Individual >>>>> Cooperative >>>>> Collaborative		
Multidisciplinary	**Interdisciplinary**	**Transdisciplinary**
A team of professionals who include representation from different disciplines (two or more) and who coordinate the contributions of each profession; they are not considered to overlap with the aim of improving care provision. Each team member can use their expertise to work independently to arrive at findings; these can be consistent or contradictory	A group of health and/or social care professionals from a range of settings working in a coordinated way towards a common goal for the person being cared for or supported. These teams work in a cooperative manner in order to succeed	A team composed of members of a number of different professions cooperating across disciplines to improve patient care through their work or research. These team members collaborate and share ideas

information to help you in your work with the people to whom you provide services; you may be able to provide useful information to support those being cared for.

Who makes up the team membership will largely depend on the purpose of the team. Each team member should be clear about their own role as well as that of every other member of the team. In understanding roles consider the purpose of the role, as well as the levels of accountability, authority and responsibility related to the role. Lack of clarity around these roles and responsibilities can lead to errors, distrust, confusion, inappropriate or no delegation, poor or inappropriate use of resources, increased stress, tendency to blame and lack of motivation.

Thinking cap 2.1

Think about what it is that you would most like other team members to know or understand about your role.

All health and social care workers must know exactly what is expected of them in their role. You have to fully understand your role and function and the ways in which you are required to work that have been agreed with those who employ you. It is important that you have good working relationships with those you offer care and support to, your colleagues in the workplace and those you work with from other agencies.

Teams and teamworking

The words 'group' and 'team' are often used interchangeably. Any team should be regarded as a group; it becomes a team once it gets organised and fulfils a purpose. Teamworking occurs when a group of people work together to accomplish something. Fully functioning, effective teams are committed to a common purpose with skills that complement each other. The group of people making up the team will have complementary skills, working in a cooperative manner.

Teams are more than just a group; they are committed to a common purpose, achieving certain goals for which they hold themselves equally accountable. Organisations have introduced teamworking in order to achieve the following:

- Develop productivity.
- Improve the quality of services or products provided.
- Enhance customer focus.
- Develop the spread of ideas.
- Make a response to opportunities and threats in fast-changing environments.
- Motivate employees.
- Bring in multi-skilling and employee flexibility.

Stop, look, respond 2.3

Teams and teamworking

Make notes and think of a team that you are a part of:

- What works well in the team?
- What doesn't always work well?
- What do individuals bring to the team?
- What roles do individuals have in the team?
- What changes would you make to the team to make it a better team?

Until the purpose of the team has been decided, it will not be able to function effectively. Agreeing on aims, objectives and goals is a key component of teamworking; this provides focus as well as strategic direction. Clarity is required as well as aims, objectives and goals but also with regards to responsibilities within the team. The team has to agree on ways in which it will judge its successes or failures.

Teams can be tight-knit units that are composed of individuals who, on a regular basis, work together; alternatively they may be ad hoc, loosely woven and only meet to address specific demands. Teams can be formally established and have a particular structure or objective, or they can just grow and come together without any formal recognition.

In health and social care the most common type of team that is spoken about is the multidisciplinary team. On a shift to shift basis there are a number of staff who are providing direct care and support and the emphasis here would be on the care and support team. The team can comprise whatever groups or levels of care and support staff are deemed appropriate to provide a safe and effective service. The composition of the team will depend on a number of factors, with an emphasis on staff availability, level of staffing and skill mix. A team should have a staff member who takes on the team leader role; team leader roles have different titles depending on your own organisation's structures. Some teams will be big and others will be small; there is no limit to how the team is to be formed so long as the formation meets the needs of those being cared for or supported.

Agreed ways of working, Codes of Conduct and contracts of employment will require you to work as a team member as well as working as individuals. Your job description will make much reference to teamwork and teamworking. You cannot work effectively as a team member unless you know what your own contribution to that team is to be, and your own strengths and limitations; you also have to be self-aware (looking inwardly). No health or social care staff should work in isolation. You are required to work with colleagues in a cooperative manner, respecting their skills, their expertise and the contribution that they make. If you know what skills and expertise others can contribute you will be able to make appropriate referrals to them. In order to work as an effective team member you must have effective communication skills.

 ## Stop, look, respond 2.4

Contributing to the team

Choose a situation that involved you and other members of the multi-professional team working together. Reflect upon your performance within the team and make notes about:

- What were my strongest features?
- What were my areas for improvement?
- How did I work with other agencies outside of the team?
- Thinking back were there any aspects of teamworking that I could have improved upon? If so, what were they and how would I have managed the situation differently?
- Are there any aspects of teamworking in which I think I need to develop? Make a list of these.

A number of high-profile failures in health and social care systems have been identified; there is a need for cooperation and collaboration between health and social care workers at all levels. A need to move towards a culture that seeks to foster mutual respect as well as shared values away from the concept of working in isolation is required.

Team dynamics

Team dynamics are invisible forces that work between different people or groups in a team. Team dynamics can have a big impact on team performance. They can have a good or a bad impact on how a team behaves or performs, and their effects can be complex. When a team underperforms the consequences can be severe, as any aspect of care provision relies on others directly or indirectly.

Team dynamics are the unconscious, psychological forces that influence the direction of a team's behaviour and performance; they are evident when the team interacts. Like undercurrents in the sea, they can carry boats in a different direction to the one they intend to sail. Team dynamics are created by the nature of the team's work, the personalities within the team, their working relationships with other people and the environment in which the team works.

Barriers to effective teamworking

For teams to work together successfully they usually have to overcome a number of barriers. The fundamental aspect of teamworking is the coming together of many minds and bodies working in unison to accomplish a common goal. Successful teams take advantage of the unique strengths

Table 2.2   Some barriers to effective teamworking

- Unclear or unproductive communication
- Different approaches result in individuals working in isolation
- The team cannot make a consensus decision when required
- The team fails to understand the other team members' roles
- The team is not clear in its aims or goals (the common goal)

and perspectives of the individuals within the team. However, often the differences themselves prevent effective communication. For teams to function effectively they have to overcome the barriers they face. Table 2.2 highlights some of these barriers.

The team has to communicate, and this means its members will have to actively listen. Repeating back what they think they have heard can allow the individual who is communicating the original idea to correct the understanding and strengthen effective communication.

It should be acknowledged within the team that individuals approach things differently. This is important so the group can understand that there are many ways to work things through. It can also provide an opportunity to appreciate each person's uniqueness and why they have approached an issue in their unique way.

It is not always appropriate for all decisions to be made through consensus but there are times when all team members should be provided with a say in order to buy in and carry the decision through. The processes by which individuals come to different decisions depend on a number of factors so consensus decisions are not always appropriate.

There may be times when not all members of the team fully understand and appreciate what the roles of the other team members are. Role clarification or review may be needed.

On occasion the common aim or goal of the team may be lost or indeed may not have been clearly defined or understood by all team members. If individuals do not understand the common goal they are less likely to contribute in an effective manner or work together as a team to accomplish the task before them. Regular review of aims and objectives and achievements can help to ensure that the group understands the goal they are trying to achieve as a team and the benefits of working together as a team.

Conflict

When people have opposing ideas, differing needs or beliefs, or a lack of knowledge about roles and responsibilities of others within the team and their values or goals, then conflict within a team is likely to occur. Conflict has positive attributes but it has to be managed otherwise it can be problematic.

Thinking cap 2.2

Think of a time when conflict has arisen within your team; how was this managed?

Conflict can be the cause of or can result in:

- power struggles;
- competition with regard to resources;

- personal resentments;
- miscommunication;
- disrespect;
- increased stress;
- decreased productivity;
- breakdown of the team (along with disengagement).

Whilst these are the negative repercussions of stress, the following can be seen as the benefits that arise out of stress:

- Promotion of growth through learning how to overcome challenges.
- Development of creativity and innovation that arise out of differences.
- Enhancement of interpersonal skills as team members endeavour to resolve issues.
- Respect and understanding.

Stop, look, respond 2.5

Conflict

In the figure below make notes about the impact that conflict might have on the various entities.

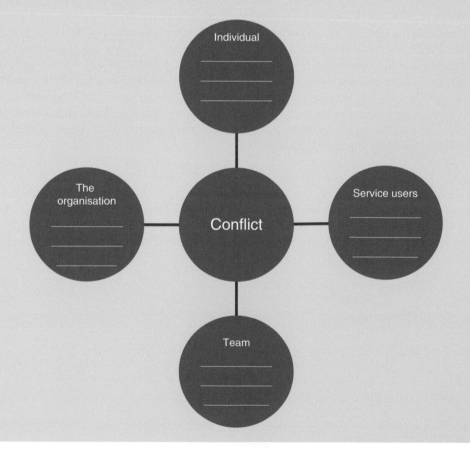

Managing conflict requires that all parties are mutually respected, conflict management should be approached with an open mind and willingness to resolve issues and, if needed, to compromise.

Chapter summary

- Teamwork is key in the provision of health and social care.
- No single person, group or professional can deliver a complete episode of health or social care.
- Teams work most effectively when they have a clear purpose, effective communication, coordination, protocols and procedures.
- An effective team understands what teamworking involves.
- A team is made up of people with different skills who share ideas, challenge one another and respect each other's contribution.
- The active participation of all members is a key feature.
- The make-up and functioning of teams will vary depending on the needs of those being cared for or supported.
- Teams function differently depending on where they operate.
- Conflict is pretty much inevitable when working with others.
- Conflict is not necessarily a bad thing.

Case scenario 2.1

Dion

Dion is a Black African American, aged 68 years, who has been experiencing a number of urinary symptoms, for example, urgency to pass urine, lower abdominal pain, getting up in the middle of the night to urinate, and blood in his urine. He had seen his general practitioner with these urinary symptoms and was referred to a consultant urologist. Dion has undergone a series of tests, which included blood tests, a physical examination, a prostatic biopsy and an ultrasound. A diagnosis was made and he has locally advanced prostate cancer.

Dion has been provided with information to help him make an informed decision. Treatment options have been provided and they include:

- Watchful waiting
- Surgery
- Radiotherapy
- Chemotherapy
- Hormone therapy
- Brachytherapy

Dion and his wife are clearly upset with this diagnosis, and the nurse has suggested that they seek counselling and further support.

From this short scenario who do you think, from a health and social care professional perspective, might Dion meet as he starts on his journey? Think about their roles and responsibilities when caring for and offering support to Dion and his family.

Resource file

Mind tools
https://www.mindtools.com
Provides a range of practical, straightforward tools to help you excel in your career.

NHS England
https://www.england.nhs.uk/wp-content/uploads/2015/01/mdt-dev-guid-flat-fin.pdf
MDT Development. An NHS publication that focuses on multidisciplinary teams.

Skills for care
http://www.skillsforcare.org.uk/Home.aspx
The employer-led workforce development body for adult social care in England.

Chapter 3

Understanding your role

Care certificate outcomes

1. Understand your own role.
2. Work in ways that have been agreed with your employer.
3. Understand working relationships in health and social care.
4. Work in partnership with others.

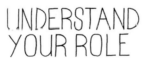

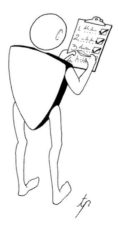

Fundamentals of Care: A Textbook for Health and Social Care Assistants, First Edition. Ian Peate.
© 2017 John Wiley & Sons Ltd. Published 2017 by John Wiley & Sons Ltd.

Take stock

Rate your current knowledge and skills prior to reading this chapter. Put a tick in the box that you think applies to you with regards to the standard being discussed:

Key:

I know this
I have a good level of knowledge or skills regarding this aspect of the standard. I make use of the knowledge and skills identified on a regular basis, feeling confident in my ability and performance. I do not need a refresher.

Satisfactory
My level of knowledge and standard of skills meet the criteria associated with the standard. I use the skills and knowledge from time to time. I might not always feel confident in my capability. I would benefit from a refresher.

I require a review
I do not feel that I have the skills and/or the knowledge that would enable me to meet the standard in a confident and competent way. The knowledge and skills I used to have are no longer valid. I will require a refresher.

This is new to me
I have never worked in a caring role before or I have never covered this topic before. I will need further training and development in this area.

Standard	Self-assessment			
Understanding your role	☐ I know this	☐ Satisfactory	☐ I should review this	☐ This is new to me
Working in ways that have been agreed with your employer	☐ I know this	☐ Satisfactory	☐ I should review this	☐ This is new to me
Understand working relationships in health and social care	☐ I know this	☐ Satisfactory	☐ I should review this	☐ This is new to me
Work with others in partnership	☐ I know this	☐ Satisfactory	☐ I should review this	☐ This is new to me
Understanding my code of conduct	☐ I know this	☐ Satisfactory	☐ I should review this	☐ This is new to me
Working in an accountable way	☐ I know this	☐ Satisfactory	☐ I should review this	☐ This is new to me

Introduction

The contribution that care workers make to the health and wellbeing of people cannot be underestimated. The ways in which care assistants work across the UK will differ as there is no one core job description for care workers. Nevertheless, each member of staff will have a job description (sometimes these can be called person specifications or role descriptors). Regardless of where you work you will have a job description.

It is essential that you understand your role and function, the ways in which you are to work that have been agreed with those who employ you. When you understand your role others should also appreciate what is expected of you; this will help in developing working relationships in health and social care, enhancing partnership working with others.

Who are you?

Your experiences, attitudes and beliefs are key attributes of who you are and we all have different experiences, attitudes and beliefs. They will have an impact (for better for worse) on how you think, what you do and how you do it.

Thinking cap 3.1

Attitudes and beliefs

Take some time to think about you. Who would you say is the person who has influenced you most in your life? Why?

Your background, the way you were reared (your upbringing), experiences and relationships will all have an influence on how you see things. Our attitudes and beliefs can lead us to make assumptions about people, and there are times when the assumptions we make are wrong.

If you are self-aware (paying attention to how you behave) you can develop ways in which you can check out if you are making erroneous assumptions about others based on wrong information or on your experiences and beliefs. Taking time to understand the diverse attitudes and beliefs that others have can help you work with them in a respectful, considerate and effective way.

Stop, look, respond 3.1

Self-awareness

Think about an occasion in practice when your feelings could have influenced your thoughts and behaviour. How did you feel? Did you feel that you were in control of the situation? And did your emotions influence your level of confidence in this situation or how you perceived others? Our emotions are powerful; they can prompt action and inaction, interaction, intervention and withdrawal.

Job description

A job description is an outline of a job. It can be anything from a few sentences to a few pages long, and it will tell you what your main duties and responsibilities are and to whom you have to report. As a care assistant you should know what is expected of you and also what is not included in your role. No job description could ever list every task that you undertake. Having said this it should, however, largely reflect the role that you are paid to do.

Stop, look, respond 3.2

Your role

Think about your current role and make a list of the various aspects of your job:

_____

_____

_____

_____

_____

Having considered the various elements of work that you do (and you should have a very long list), can you group the work under the following headings:

- Providing care and support
- Working as part of a team
- Contributing to activities
- Respecting confidentiality

Stop, look, respond 3.3

The job description

Retrieve a copy of your current job description (your manager will have a copy if you do not).

1. What is the purpose of the position? (The reasons for the position's existence)

    _____

    _____

    _____

    _____

    _____

2. What is the position? (Title, grade/salary, department, directorate and so on)

    _____

    _____

    _____

    _____

    _____

3. What are the essential functions associated with the position? (The tasks critical to the position)

    _____

    _____

    _____

    _____

    _____

4. Periodic functions? (Tasks that are not essential, but are part of the job description)
_____
_____
_____
_____

5. List the minimum qualifications? (Education, experience)

_____
_____
_____
_____

6. What are the required behaviours? (Attention to detail, ability to learn, knowledge, skills, attitude)
_____
_____
_____
_____

7. Describe the working conditions (Description of the physical requirements, environmental issues)
_____
_____
_____
_____
_____
_____

8. Any supervision needed? (How the job is supervised, whether you are expected to work independently)
_____
_____
_____
_____
_____
_____
_____

9. Miscellaneous: 'Other tasks as assigned' – What might these be?
_____
_____
_____
_____
_____
_____
_____

Having scrutinised your job description, are you more aware of the role you perform and what is being asked of you? You should only carry out those tasks that are agreed in your job description and for which you are competent.

Agreed ways of working

Working in a person-centred way, communicating effectively, building relationships, and respecting equality and diversity mean that you will also have to be familiar with how the other people you work with carry out their duties. Working as part of a team requires that you are a supportive team member and that you develop your skills to improve the way you work. You must also demonstrate that you are following agreed ways of working, and adhering to regulations and rules. This will entail contributing to activities in a number of ways with the key aim of working in a safe way and respecting confidentiality.

Thinking cap 3.2

Your skills

Think about your work and how you function. Do you think you are a valued member of your organisation? Give some thought to the rationale for the answer that you have provided.

All employers will have aims and objectives that set out what their purpose is. Sometimes this can be called the mission statement or the philosophy. It is important that you are aware of what these are because as you are working for the organisation, you will be expected to adopt these aims and objectives, seeking to achieve and exceed them as you go about your work.

Stop, look, respond 3.4

Mission statement, philosophy, aims and objectives

Seek out your organisation's aims and objectives. Take some time to think about the way you work and if you are working in a way that mirrors these aims and objectives. Do you need to reassess the way you work to ensure that you are working in sync with your employer's expectations?

The organisation's aims and objectives should be revisited regularly and when attending supervision sessions and appraisals. If you have any uncertainties or doubts concerning your organisation's aims and objectives, then you should be asking your line manager for clarification.

Policies and procedures

As well as the aims and objectives, the organisation will also have a variety of policies and procedures. These should incorporate relevant laws and legislation that will help to support you as you deliver care in a safe and effective manner; the policies and procedures are seen as best practice.

It is not expected that you will know every word of every policy; however, it is expected that you know what policies exist and what they are about. You should familiarise yourself with policies and procedures.

Stop, look, respond 3.5

Policies and procedures

In your place of work look for a policy or procedure that relates to your everyday practice. Most polices follow a format. Identify the following from the policy you have chosen:

Where is the policy kept (paper copy or on the intranet)?	
What is the name of the policy?	
Who prepared it?	
When was it prepared (effective date) and when is it due for review (revision)?	
What is the purpose of the policy?	
Who is it applicable to (practice level competency/target audience)?	
What is the procedure (how to do it; how to meet the policy requirements and the goals)?	
Who is responsible for implementing it?	

If you fail to adhere to agreed ways of working, policies or procedures then you are in danger of harming the people you care for, the people you work with and yourself. Further, you could find yourself subject to capability or disciplinary procedures by your employer, and this may lead to dismissal or prosecution.

Thinking cap 3.3

Policy and procedures

Think about the advantages of having policies and procedures in your workplace. Think about this from your perspective and also from the perspective of the people you offer care to and those with whom you work.

Do you think there are any disadvantages associated with the use of policies and procedures?

Codes of conduct

Where you are in the UK and in what sphere you are employed will reflect which Codes of Conduct you are working within:

- Skills for Care/Skills for Health have published a Code of Conduct for Health Care Support Workers and Adult Social Care Workers in England.
- The Scottish Social Services Council has published Codes of Practice for Social Service Workers and Employers.

- The Social Care Council in Northern Ireland has a Code of Practice for Social Care Workers and Employers of Social Care Workers.
- The Care Council for Wales has a Code of Practice for Social Care Workers.

An employer may also have a Code of Conduct or a directive (a policy) in place that guides the care worker regarding the use and the application of the Codes. You will also have a contract of employment that can also be seen as a code requiring you to work in agreed ways.

Some Social Care Councils require you to register with them as a practitioner or supervisor, and in so doing you will agree to adhere to their Codes of Conduct or practice, just as other registered healthcare practitioners have to, for example a social worker, physiotherapist or nurse. Failure to comply with these directives may result in referral to the organisation and fitness to practice or conduct and competency hearings. Some Social Care Workers can also be removed from the register in the same way that any other registered health and care practitioner can.

The various Codes of Conduct provide the moral and ethical standards that are expected of all health and social care workers.

Stop, look, respond 3.6

Codes of conduct

1. Choose a code of conduct that you work to. Read the code and write notes related to the various subheadings.

    _____
    _____
    _____
    _____
    _____
    _____
    _____

2. Make a list of your responsibilities as a healthcare support worker or adult social care worker.

    _____
    _____
    _____
    _____
    _____
    _____

The employer is required to tell you the safe and agreed ways in which you are expected to work. This can be shared with you as part of a particular policy, or your manager or another colleague may provide this in person. Agreed ways of working with each individual will be provided in care plans; these ensure that you are working within the law and you are providing care and support that reflects the needs of the person you are providing care to. If you fail to follow the agreed ways of working then there is a possibility that you could harm yourself or others. You are responsible for your own work, and if people suffer harm as a result of your actions then you may face disciplinary procedures. The outcome could lead to dismissal or prosecution.

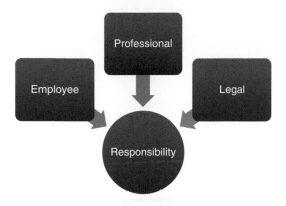

Figure 3.1   Three intertwined aspects of responsibility.

Responsibility

You have a number of responsibilities to the people for whom you are providing care and support. It is your responsibility that:

- Their safety and wellbeing are protected, and that their care plan is adhered to and is carried out in an agreed and safe way.
- The care that you provide meets each individual's needs by involving them and their carer(s) or support network when care is planned, reviewed and delivered.
- They are treated fairly and that you promote equality and diversity and respect their dignity and human rights.

Responsibility can be seen as a set of tasks that an employer, professional body, court of law or some other recognised body can reasonably demand. Responsibility can be considered from three aspects (Figure 3.1); all three aspects are intertwined and they do not function in isolation.

Employee responsibilities

Employee responsibilities are often outlined in the contract of employment and the job description; these set out in detail what the individual responsibilities of an employee are. The responsibilities outlined should be revised and regularly revisited, formally and informally, as part of an individual's ongoing appraisal. Employee responsibilities are closely aligned to the work objectives of the individual, of the team and of the organisation.

Professional responsibilities

Often these are defined by the duty of care owed to the service user, professional codes of conduct, registration and regulation. Employees must recognise and appreciate the limits of their own knowledge and competence. It is also just as important to ensure that anyone they delegate to has the required knowledge and competence in order to carry out the delegated task.

Legal responsibilities

Legal responsibilities are part of Codes of Conduct as these are often derived from law. Each care worker has an obligation to comply with the laws and legislation of the country in which they work (the four countries of the UK often have legislation that is country specific).

Stop, look, respond 3.7

Responsibility

Make notes and give work examples regarding the three different types of responsibility.

Types of responsibility	Notes and examples
Employee	
Professional	
Legal	

Accountability

Accountability means being answerable to oneself and others for your own actions. In order for you to be accountable, you must act in accordance with your code of conduct. You will be accountable for any judgments made and actions that you take in the course of your practice.

You may be called upon to provide an explanation, to clarify, or give a reason for why you did something in a particular way (being called to account). The same would apply if you did not do something (if you omitted to do something). It is not acceptable to say 'I was just following orders'; in law being ignorant is no defence. Being aware of what accountability is and what it is not can help you to expand and develop your practice when making safe and effective responses to those you offer care to. It is acknowledged that accountability is not responsibility; however, they are very closely linked.

The Code of Conduct for Health Care Support Workers and Adult Social Care Workers in England (2013) states that:

> as a Healthcare Support Worker or Adult Social Care Worker in England you must be accountable by making sure you can answer for your actions or omissions

Being accountable requires you to be honest with yourself and others regarding what you can and cannot do, appreciating your abilities and any limitations related to your sphere of competence. You should only undertake those tasks that have been agreed in your job description and for which you are competent.

You have to act and present yourself in such a way that your suitability to work in a health or social care environment is not called into question. Be able to justify and be answerable (be accountable) for your actions or your omissions. If you do not feel able to or are not prepared to carry out any aspect of work then seek guidance. Inform those supervising you or your employer about any issues that could impact on your ability to carry out your job competently and safely.

Build up and support clear and appropriate professional boundaries in relationships that you have with those who use health and care services, carers and colleagues. You must not accept any offers of loans, gifts, benefits or hospitality from anyone you are offering support to or anyone close to them that could be seen to compromise your position.

Adhere to agreed ways of working. Report any actions or omissions by yourself or colleagues that you suspect could possibly compromise the safety or care of those who use health and care services. You must if required use whistle-blowing procedures in order to report any suspected wrongdoing.

Delegation

Delegation can be described as the passing of work or tasks from one person to another. Delegation is the process by which a person (the delegator) allocates clinical or non-clinical treatment or care to a competent person (the delegatee). There are, however, certain issues that have to be taken into consideration prior to delegating (Table 3.1).

Before you accept a task that has been delegated to you, you should remember that you are responsible and accountable for ensuring that your knowledge and skills are up to date. You must work within the guidelines and protocols of the organisation. Ensure that your job description permits you to accept the delegated activity. Ensure that your job description is checked and updated regularly in order to reflect changes in tasks and responsibilities. Know what it is that you have to do if you have any concerns that relate to the delegated task you are being asked to perform, and know who it is you have to ask for advice or support.

Stop, look, respond 3.8

Delegated activities

Provide a list of ten examples of work that has been delegated to you.

1. _____
2. _____
3. _____
4. _____
5. _____
6. _____
7. _____
8. _____
9. _____
10. _____

Table 3.1   Considerations prior to delegating

- The best interests of the service user
- The clinical risk perceived in delegating the task
- The required task
- The work capacity of the person being required to complete the task
- The knowledge of the person being asked to undertake the task
- The confidence and competence of the person being asked to complete the task
- The benefit for the person who accepts the delegated task

The decision as to which activities are suitable to delegate rests with the person delegating; there is no nationally available specific guidance regarding the activities that can or cannot be delegated. In general the law does not dictate who might perform particular care tasks or undertake specific roles.

Stop, look, respond 3.9

Delegation

Write some notes about the following commonly used terms in delegation:

Accountability	
Appropriate	
Capability	
Capacity	
Competence	
Competencies	
Competent	
Consent	
Delegate	
Delegatee	
Delegation	
Delegator	
Performance	
Policy	
Protocol	
Reliable	
Responsible	
Supervision	
Task	

Relationships

Those working as healthcare support workers are privileged in the relationships they have with those they offer care to. But this also brings with it a professional duty of care to the service users. This is a very different relationship to any relationship a person may have with their friends and family.

Table 3.2   Strategies that can help you to maintain professional boundaries

- Understand local policy and procedure
- Be clear about your role
- Respect the person as an individual
- Be aware of the potential power imbalance
- Ensure you keep your personal life private
- Only use appropriate body contact
- Make appropriate use of chaperones
- Use gloves when carrying out intimate procedures, for example, when examining the genitalia
- Discuss with the person issues concerning sexual boundaries if there is a possibility that they have been or may be crossed

The key elements of the care worker's role are to offer guidance, provide care and to support service users in helping them to live as they choose to, doing this by respecting their choices, and carefully listening without making judgments or prejudice.

Many service users to whom you provide care and offer support will be vulnerable, and they will expect you to follow policy, protocol and procedure. These can help to ensure that your professional boundaries and relationships will be maintained. The care worker must not form inappropriate intimate or personal relationships with people they care for. You have a duty to promote an individual's independence and protect them as far as possible from harm.

Do not accept gifts or money from individuals or their family members, and be honest and trustworthy. If you have any concerns then report these to your line manager.

Table 3.2 outlines strategies that can help you to maintain professional boundaries.

 Stop, look, respond 3.10

Relationships

Take some time and consider how your relationships with service users differ from those with your friends and family. Write your thoughts down in the boxes below and compare them.

Service users	Family and friends

Chapter summary

- Understanding your role and those with whom you work can only help you to advance the quality of care that you provide.
- Your unique life experiences, the attitudes you have and beliefs you hold are central components of who you are. It must be acknowledged that each one of us, those who provide and those to whom we provide care, all have different experiences, attitudes and beliefs.
- As a care provider it is important that you understand what is expected of you so you are able to practise safely and effectively, ensure you are not harming those you care for, yourself or the people you work with. Your job description provides information regarding your role. However, no job description could ever list every task you undertake; it will, however, generally reflect the role you are paid to do.
- Employers have aims and objectives that express what their purpose is (sometimes called the mission statement or the philosophy). You should make yourself familiar with these aims and objectives, demonstrating that you are following agreed ways of working. You will be expected to adopt these aims and objectives, seeking to achieve and exceed them as you go about your work.
- The organisation where you work will also have a variety of policies and procedures as well as its aims and objectives. Policies and procedures incorporate relevant laws and legislation, helping to support you as you deliver care in a safe and effective manner; they are seen as best practice.
- Where you work in the UK and in what area of work you are employed will reflect which Codes of Conduct you are required to adhere to. An employer may also have a Code of Conduct or a directive guiding the care worker with regards to the use and the application of the Codes. Your contract of employment can also be seen as a code requiring you to work in agreed ways.
- Responsibility can be considered from three aspects – professional, legal and employee. All three aspects are intertwined; they do not function in isolation.
- Accountability, just like responsibility, is complex; it means being answerable to oneself and to others for your own actions and omissions.
- You may be called upon to provide an explanation, to clarify, or give a reason for why you did something in a particular way just as if you did not do something (if you omitted to do something). It is unacceptable to say 'I was just following orders'. Accountability is not the same as responsibility; however, they are very closely linked.
- Before you take on a task that has been delegated to you, you must remember that you are responsible and accountable for guaranteeing that your knowledge and skills are up to date. You have to work within the guidelines and protocols of the organisation, ensuring that your job description permits you to accept the delegated activity.

 ## Case scenario 3.1

Folami

Folami works as an activities worker in a dementia care centre. Folami is assisting the occupational therapist (Jay), and Jay and Folami have worked together for a number of years. The occupational therapist has set up a range of activities for a group of six people he is working with. The aim of the session is to enhance function, promote relationships and social participation, and to find ways for those members of the group to enjoy life. One member of the group, Marie, becomes disorientated and tends to wander; preserving Marie's safety is a key issue.

Jay receives a telephone call to say that his son has had a fall in the playground at school and the child is on his way to the local accident and emergency department. Jay is clearly upset by the telephone call; he asks Folami to supervise the group whilst he goes to the accident and emergency department to be with his son. Folami is not happy with this request.

What might be your reaction to a request by a registered practitioner who asks you to undertake an activity or to respond to a request that you know you are not competent to perform?
Who might you turn to if you found yourself in a similar situation?

Resource file

Skills for Care/Skills for Health have published a Code of Conduct for Health Care Support Workers and Adult Social Care Workers in England
http://www.skillsforhealth.org.uk/images/services/code-of-conduct/Code%20of%20Conduct%20Healthcare%20Support.pdf

Scottish Social Services Council have published Codes of Practice for Social Service Workers and Employers
http://www.sssc.uk.com/about-the-sssc/multimedia-library/publications/60-protecting-the-public/61-codes-of-practice/1020-sssc-codes-of-practice-for-social-service-workers-and-employers

The Northern Ireland Social Care Council has a Code of Practice for Employers of Social Care Workers
http://www.niscc.info/storage/resources/20151118_codesforemployers_updated.pdf

The Care Council for Wales has a Code of Professional Practice for Social Care Workers
http://www.ccwales.org.uk/code-of-professional-practice/

Chapter 4

Your personal development

Care certificate outcomes

1. Agree a personal development plan.
2. Develop your knowledge, skills and understanding.

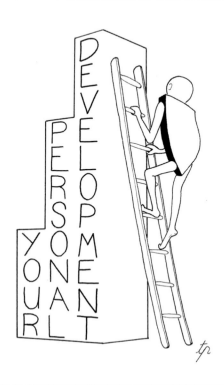

Fundamentals of Care: A Textbook for Health and Social Care Assistants, First Edition. Ian Peate.
© 2017 John Wiley & Sons Ltd. Published 2017 by John Wiley & Sons Ltd.

Take stock

Rate your current knowledge and skills prior to reading this chapter. Put a tick in the box that you think applies to you with regards to the standard being discussed:

Key:

I know this
I have a good level of knowledge or skills regarding this aspect of the standard. I make use of the knowledge and skills identified on a regular basis, feeling confident in my ability and performance. I do not need a refresher.

Satisfactory
My level of knowledge and standard of skills meet the criteria associated with the standard. I use the skills and knowledge from time to time. I might not always feel confident in my capability. I would benefit from a refresher.

I require a review
I do not feel that I have the skills and/or the knowledge that would enable me to meet the standard in a confident and competent way. The knowledge and skills I used to have are no longer valid. I will require a refresher.

This is new to me
I have never worked in a caring role before or I have never covered this topic before. I will need further training and development in this area.

Standard	Self-assessment			
Appreciate the value of lifelong learning	☐ I know this	☐ Satisfactory	☐ I should review this	☐ This is new to me
Aware of my learning style	☐ I know this	☐ Satisfactory	☐ I should review this	☐ This is new to me
Understand the importance of the personal development plan	☐ I know this	☐ Satisfactory	☐ I should review this	☐ This is new to me
Understanding of the annual appraisal process	☐ I know this	☐ Satisfactory	☐ I should review this	☐ This is new to me
Appreciate the need for a personal development portfolio	☐ I know this	☐ Satisfactory	☐ I should review this	☐ This is new to me
Aware of my training and development needs	☐ I know this	☐ Satisfactory	☐ I should review this	☐ This is new to me

Introduction

The quality of care provided to people is profoundly influenced by the performance of individual health and care workers. In order to remain competent you must remain up to date with regards to your knowledge and skills. This a key feature of your personal development, and this has to be continual – lifelong. You need to be ready to acknowledge 'not knowing'. This is a prerequisite if you are to be committed to learning and committed to doing something about it. One of the pillars in advancing care is to ensure that those who are providing care are prepared in such a way that this reflects 21st century health and social care provision.

Personal development is also linked to continuous professional development (CPD) or continuing personal and professional development (CPPD). Lifelong learning is a key element of personal development.

Lifelong learning

In order to keep up to date and to ensure that the care and support offered are responsive to needs, the whole workforce has to be prepared for changing health and social care practices and treatments. If staff are not adequately prepared then the standard and the quality of care provided to people will not progress. Lifelong learning is important as what we learn in health and social care can very quickly become out of date. Lifelong learning:

- can result in better care planning;
- generates an exchange of ideas between staff and those who use our services;
- helps to motivate staff; and
- can develop confidence and competence.

Your lifelong learning forms a part of your personal development plan (PDP). Lifelong learning can be described as a continuum of health- and care-related education and training from commencing practice as a heath or care worker to retirement. Lifelong learning links health and care education with the delivery of care within the workplace; it is one form of continuing education.

How learning takes place, learning styles

The skills you learn and the knowledge you gain can be put into practice immediately for career advancement and can provide lifelong value. A positive learning environment will improve the quality of care.

Those who provide care and offer support to others bring with them a range of experiences and qualities; one element of this is their diverse learning styles, their individual learning preferences. Learning styles are particular to an individual; recognising and acknowledging these can help a person to learn. All of us have some particular preferred method of interacting with and processing the vast amounts of information we are continually receiving.

There are over 70 different published models that relate to learning styles. They tend to focus on different aspects such as cognitive processes (our thought processes), personality descriptions, talents, how we perceive (sense) things, learning processes and thinking styles. The various theories of learning styles agree that we do not all learn in the same way; we learn in different ways and at different levels, both as individuals and in groups.

Peter Honey and Alan Mumford have identified four separate learning styles or preferences:

1. Activist
2. Theorist
3. Pragmatist
4. Reflector

These are the learning approaches that people are said to naturally prefer. Once you have identified your learning style and you have sought out opportunities to learn using that style then you will have the potential to maximise your own personal learning.

Stop, look, respond 4.1

Learning styles

There are many websites available that will enable you to find out your preferred learning style(s). This one provides further information about Honey and Mumford's learning styles: http://www.brainboxx.co.uk/a2_learnstyles/pages/learningstyles.htm

The questionnaires can assist in identifying your learning preferences. Then you will be better positioned to choose learning opportunities that suit your style.

What was your preferred learning style(s)?

Strategies to help with learning

The VARK questionnaire helps your learning by suggesting the strategies you should be using in order to get the most out of your learning. VARK stands for:

Visual
Auditory
Reading/writing
Kinaesthetic

The four areas are referred to as modalities and they inform you as to how best you process information. Knowing the mode best suited to you (there may be more than one mode) can help you improve the way you study.

A person who learns better using the visual mode prefers looking at pictures, watching videos and graphs, and using highlighters and symbols. Aural (auditory or hearing) learners are said to learn better when they are part of a discussion group, using recordings, maybe podcasts; they enjoy telling their ideas to other people. A read-and-write learner prefers to list things, read out of textbooks, handouts, and using a highlighter; these learners often take a large amount of notes. A kinaesthetic person learns better when undertaking hands-on activities, for example, project work.

Now you have some idea of your preferred learning style and the approach to learning that best suits you, you are ideally placed to build upon the current strategies that you currently use.

Stop, look, respond 4.2

Strategies

There are many websites available that will enable you to identify your preferred learning style. They often use adapted versions of VARK; you should search the websites. This website uses VAK (visual, auditory and kinaesthetic) and it is free, just follow the instructions:
http://www.businessballs.com/vaklearningstylestest.htm

So, which modality best suits you?

Thinking cap 4.1

Using self-assessment tools

What are some of the drawbacks/cautions associated with using self-assessment tools?
   Remember they are only guides to the mixture of preferences, strengths and learning styles in an individual, and cannot be used as a basis for deciding on one exclusive preference or approach to the exclusion of everything else.

Personal development plans

In order to improve your knowledge and skills you will need to embrace, value and embed personal development activities as a lifelong process. You will be able to:

- Demonstrate a growth in confidence.
- Demonstrate a professional approach to the ways in which you work.
- Take on responsibility for your own continuing professional and personal development.
- Express a willingness to take part in the development of others.
- Demonstrate increasing confidence and competence.
- Share your knowledge with others.
- Recognise the importance of statutory and mandatory training.

You will also be able to demonstrate good time management and organisational skills.

Your personal development plan (PDP) is just that – yours; you must take ownership of this very important activity. PDPs can permeate our lives at work; however, this is a little different; PDPs can help in a number of ways – they can be used for short- and long-term planning.

Your PDP can be seen as an action plan that will assist you in getting organised, ensuring that you have the necessary skills and knowledge when opportunities to progress arise. The PDP, if undertaken in a systematic and ordered way, will identify the learning and development needs that you require in order to help you perform your job better. It then sets the baseline from where you progress and your progression can be tracked.

As is the case with such action plans, this is intended to help you bring about change. In this instance this should be directed specifically at improving your readiness and effectiveness to provide safe, effective and person-centred care.

Personal development plans can be formulated for a number of reasons; one of the most common is after the annual appraisal has taken place. PDPs can also emerge as a result of induction for new staff or for those staff who are changing roles.

Appraisal

Appraisal (sometimes called individual performance review, job evaluation or personal development planning) is a one-to-one meeting. This is a formal forum where the review takes place. The aim is to encourage and motivate people to perform at their maximum potential, and it is an essential component of career development. The appraisal process should be an open dialogue between the member of staff and their manager (it is usually the manager who undertakes the appraisal). It also allows for protected time for a discussion of personal development in the person's role, their career development aspirations and service provision. Your manager is responsible for arranging the appraisal, and will inform you when and where the appraisal is to take place.

Preparing for appraisal

Preparation is the most important activity that can be undertaken when being appraised. It is important that you are familiar with the core and specific dimensions associated with your role and the purpose of the appraisal. It is essential to be clear about your role because the key aims and goals of both the place where you work and the area in which you work will be a focus of the appraisal and the objectives that will be set following it. In preparing ensure that you are fully conversant with your job/role description.

Arrive in good time for the appraisal so that you are not flustered or hurried. If you are required to bring any documentation with you be sure you have it. The appraisal process is a two-way process, and the person who is undertaking your appraisal should also have prepared for the event.

The appraisal meeting

The purpose is to provide an opportunity to have a constructive discussion with your manager about your work and how you have performed over the past year, the progress you are making and any future needs that you might have related to how you work. There should be an opportunity to discuss what has gone well during the year. Any previously agreed objectives will be discussed, and during the meeting you may identify issues that may be done differently next year. You will also be provided with the opportunity to identify obstacles that might have prevented you from achieving your objectives, and to agree ways forward.

The completion of an appraisal should culminate in agreed future objectives that have been set with a clear link to the area where you work, incorporating the area's plans and aspirations as well as the organisation's overall strategic direction.

Thinking cap 4.2

Appraisal

Who would you turn to if you felt that during your appraisal you were treated unfairly?

Your personal development plan

A personal developmental plan will be prepared to help you meet the agreed objectives decided upon during appraisal. The plan will detail what your role is in achieving these objectives and the support that the organisation will offer. The support that is needed might be, for example, the identification of training or developmental needs. You will be asked how you will achieve the objectives, what role you will play and your long-term career aspirations. These must be matched to the aims and aspiration of the service in which you are working and the organisation's strategic objectives.

Agreeing your objectives

Your objectives have to spell out what it is that you want to achieve; therefore it is important to get the writing of objectives correct. Using a SMART goal system to help you write objectives can help ensure they are realistic and achievable (Figure 4.1).

SMART stands for:

- **S**pecific
- **M**easurable
- **A**chievable
- **R**elevant
- **T**ime-based

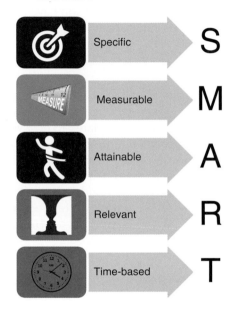

Figure 4.1   A SMART goal system.

Setting clear objectives is only one part of the process. The next stage is to break them down into manageable action points. All stages of the process should be recorded in your personal development portfolio. Included in your personal development plan must be any statutory or mandatory training that you are required to undertake by law.

The personal development portfolio

Being able to show what it is that you have achieved is a key element of the appraisal process, and putting together and maintaining a personal development portfolio is one way of doing this. There are many variations of a portfolio. In essence it should be a collation of evidence that demonstrates your achievements and is presented at the annual review meeting. The content should be:

- Valid: it provides all the appropriate information related to your job.
- Authentic: it belongs to you.
- Sufficient: there is enough evidence to demonstrate achievements.
- Current: it is up to date and appropriate reflecting the work that you do.
- Reliable: it reflects the knowledge and skills that you need to do your job.

There are many ways of collecting the required evidence. How you do this is up to you. However, your employer may have a specific way they require you to conform to. Any evidence provided must be compliant with data protection and adhere to the rules governing confidentiality. The names of people cared for and their families must be removed. Examples of evidence that can be used in a portfolio are identified in Table 4.1.

Supervision

You are responsible for collecting the evidence. However, this does not prevent you from asking your manager for support. In some organisations a more senior member of staff may supervise you. Supervision provides you with an opportunity to discuss your performance and development, talking through any aspect of your work, your role, or the people you provide care and support for. Supervision can take place one-to-one with your manager or in a group or team meeting. Regular supervisions are helpful so concerns can be addressed, progress checked and additional support provided. Table 4.2 provides a checklist that can help you to get the most out of your appraisal.

Table 4.1   Some examples of evidence that can be included in a personal development portfolio

- Information from current formal learning, for example QCF training
- Your reflective diary
- Minutes from meetings
- Written statements from others (e.g. your manager) based on direct observation of day-to-day activities
- Certificates awarded
- Training logs
- Learning and development plans (from your previous appraisal)

Table 4.2   The appraisal checklist

Before the appraisal

- Know the date and time for the appraisal
- Familiarise yourself with the venue where the appraisal is to take place
- Know about the process involved. Sometimes a self-appraisal document is needed
- Know your job description
- Assess your performance against the objectives set
- Know the strategic direction as well as the aims and objectives of the care area in which you work
- Consider what development needs you may require for the coming year
- Be sure to have all the appropriate documentation with you

During the appraisal

- Take notes if needed
- Seek clarification of any points if needed
- Be sure you understand the purpose and process
- Be confident and competent when asked about your performance
- State clearly your strengths
- Be ready to review and defend the evidence prepared
- Think about what might be done differently next year
- Be honest about any weaknesses and limitations, seeking realistic support from the manager
- Communicate effectively: listen actively and be aware of your body language and that of your manager
- Ask questions
- Check any agreement that has been made, seeking clarification if required
- Summarise and check again the agreements made, ensuring you fully understand
- Ask for clarification concerning the process for the completion and signing of any documentation
- Ask other questions if needed

Table 4.2 (Continued)

After the appraisal
• Be sure that you receive the agreements and actions from the meeting in writing
• Make comments if needed (within the agreed time span)
• If required, ask for a follow-up meeting
• Note interim review dates in your diary
• Ensure that those responsible (including yourself) take action as identified in the PDP

Ongoing activity
• Regularly speak with your manager/supervisor informally and formally about your performance and development
• Raise training and development activities at team meetings
• Review your learning activities and evaluate their effectiveness
• Continue to gather evidence for the next appraisal cycle
• Promote your own self-development and achievements
• Request and give constructive feedback

Table 4.3 Some training and development opportunities

• Shadowing another member of staff at work
• Providing mentoring or coaching to others
• Open or distance learning; private study
• Secondment to other areas or departments
• Vocational training
• Attending workshops that take place in your work place
• Guided reading: journals, books or policies
• External training opportunities
• Attending appropriate conferences
• Becoming involved in project work
• Attending meetings
• Provision of appropriate additional responsibility
• Learning from others

Training and development

Training and development opportunities are plentiful; they are not necessarily always met through attendance of a course. They can be varied, innovative and creative, with the aim of promoting lifelong learning. Creative learning and development activities can help to stimulate and encourage staff. Table 4.3 gives some examples of training and development opportunities.

Core learning

There are several core learning skills that you must have, and you must continue to develop these in order to ensure that the care you provide is safe and effective.

Regardless of where you work, you require the right level of literacy, numeracy and communication skills as you may be required to read and contribute to care plans, record information in a clear and legible way, complete forms, write emails or take notes. There will be a need for you to read and understand instructions about your ways of working. You could, for example, be involved in supporting an individual to monitor their blood pressure and you may need to keep a record of the readings and then provide this information to another healthcare worker who, based on the information you have given them, may make changes to that person's care.

Stop, look, respond 4.3

Sources of support for learning and development

There are various sources of support available to you that can help you in progressing your learning and development in your work. Identify some of the sources of support that you could use or access. These can be material resources (such as textbooks) or human resources (such as expert patients).

Resource	Description	Human or material?

Thinking cap 4.3

Learning and development

What are the barriers that might impact on your ability to learn and develop? Think of barriers within yourself and externally. How might you overcome these potential barriers?

There may be instances when you might need to understand the difference between a number of different measures, such as grams and milligrams, and be able to calculate simple conversions. Exchanging information will improve your understanding of a person's needs. If this information is incorrect or misleading then errors are likely, which can result in care provision that fails to meet the individual's care needs. Effective communication in various forms underpins all aspects of your work.

Stop, look, respond 4.4

Skillswise adult learners

Help with improving your English and maths is available via a BBC website:
http://www.bbc.co.uk/skillswise/learners

This website can help to boost your English (reading, writing, spelling, grammar and more) and also provides you with an opportunity to brush up on your maths (numbers, calculations, percentages, measuring and more).

Giving and receiving feedback

Another important aspect of your role and function is the ability to give and receive feedback; it is essential to the success of any workplace relationship.

Stop, look, respond 4.5

Feedback

Think about a time when you were given feedback, for example, at school, during an annual appraisal, when you did something really well or when you did not do something well.

How did you feel? How involved did you feel in the feedback process? Did you self-assess your own skills prior to being given feedback? Did you understand the feedback that was given to you? Did you learn about yourself and your skills because of the feedback?

Were any changes made to the way you worked following the feedback?

What was it about the way the feedback was delivered that you remembered most?

Not receiving any feedback can lead to a false assessment of our abilities. Providing constructive feedback is one way of helping to develop your confidence and your ability to solve problems as you work alongside others in the health and social care sector. Your work involves using knowledge, skills and understanding together to manage often complicated and stressful situations in a caring and compassionate manner. Receiving feedback is a key part of learning and development that will help you to develop an awareness of your strengths and those areas that require improvement.

Table 4.4 provides insight into some of the principles of feedback.

Table 4.4   Some of the principles of helpful feedback

- Plan carefully for any formal feedback session irrespective of whether you are the recipient or the provider
- Take time to think about the content of the information you are going to provide during the feedback session
- Feedback should be specific and to the point
- The feedback should focus on the issue and not on the person
- Consider the timing of your feedback session. Plan it so that both parties have a chance to benefit from the experience
- Generally, positive feedback should outweigh negative feedback

Thinking cap 4.4

Feedback

Think about how you might improve your skills with regards to the provision of feedback to others.

Feedback can be provided formally or informally. Formal feedback is often provided in written format, for example, the feedback you receive after your appraisal or the feedback given to you after you have completed an assignment. Informal feedback happens on a day-to-day basis when having discussions with work colleagues, your supervisor or those you offer care and support to and their families.

Chapter summary

- A key feature of competence and continuing personal development is a person's capacity to learn.
- Lifelong learning can be defined as a continuum of health- and care-related education and training from your beginning as a health or care worker to your retirement.
- Learning styles are particular to an individual; we all have some particular preferred method of interacting with and processing the vast amounts of information we are continually receiving.
- Your personal development plan can be seen as an action plan assisting you in getting organised, ensuring you have the necessary skills and knowledge when opportunities to progress arise.
- The appraisal is a one-to-one meeting between you and your manager reviewing how well you are working and making progress.
- A personal development portfolio contains the evidence required to demonstrate skills helping you to structure your efforts to improve in the most appropriate areas.
- Creative learning and development activities can help to stimulate and encourage.

 ## Case scenario 4.1

Jason

Jason Ketch is a domiciliary care worker providing care to people with learning disabilities who still live in their own homes. Some people require additional support with carrying out household tasks, attending to their personal care and other activities that allow them to maintain their independence and quality of life.

This is the first time that Jason has had an appraisal. Abioye, a social worker he works with (his supervisor), tells him not to worry about the appraisal, it is only a paper exercise and really no one takes it seriously.

Jason arrives late for the appraisal as it is being held in the premises of the local authority as opposed to Jason's workplace; he assumed it was being held in the resident's home. The appraisal lasted for around an hour, making Jason late for his shift as he was expecting the whole process to be over in ten minutes.

Back in the resident's home where he works he was clearly baffled by what he has just been through, explaining to Abioye that the process was much more formal than he had been led to believe. The next steps for Jason are to formally construct a PDP, but he cannot remember most of what was said during the appraisal.

He asks Abioye for his support and guidance.

In this scenario it is clear that Jason has failed to prepare himself for the appraisal. How might you ensure that you are prepared for your appraisal in order to make the most out of this activity?

Resource file

The NHS Knowledge and Skills Framework (NHS KSF)
http://www.ksf.scot.nhs.uk/uploads/documents/A_Short_Guide_to_KSF_Dimensions.pdf

Learning and the NHS Knowledge & Skills Framework (KSF) (Scotland)
http://www.vqfinder.nes.scot.nhs.uk/learning-providers/learning-and-the-nhs-knowledge--skills-framework-(ksf).aspx

Scottish Vocational Qualifications
http://www.sqa.org.uk/sqa/1514.1637.html

Qualification and Credit Framework Skills for Health
http://www.skillsforhealth.org.uk/standards/item/221-adult-vocational-qualifications-and-the-qualifications-and-credit-framework-qcf

Chapter 5

Duty of care

Care certificate outcomes

1. Understand how duty of care contributes to safe practice.
2. Understand the support available for addressing dilemmas that may arise about duty of care.
3. Deal with comments, complaints and compliments.
4. Deal with incidents, errors and near misses.
5. Deal with confrontation and difficult situations.

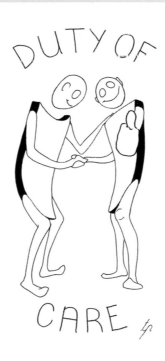

Fundamentals of Care: A Textbook for Health and Social Care Assistants, First Edition. Ian Peate.
© 2017 John Wiley & Sons Ltd. Published 2017 by John Wiley & Sons Ltd.

Take stock

Rate your current knowledge and skills prior to reading this chapter. Put a tick in the box that you think applies to you with regards to the standard being discussed:

Key:
I know this I have a good level of knowledge or skills regarding this aspect of the standard. I make use of the knowledge and skills identified on a regular basis, feeling confident in my ability and performance. I do not need a refresher.
Satisfactory My level of knowledge and standard of skills meet the criteria associated with the standard. I use the skills and knowledge from time to time. I might not always feel confident in my capability. I would benefit from a refresher.
I require a review I do not feel that I have the skills and/or the knowledge that would enable me to meet the standard in a confident and competent way. The knowledge and skills I used to have are no longer valid. I will require a refresher.
This is new to me I have never worked in a caring role before or I have never covered this topic before. I will need further training and development in this area.

Standard	Self-assessment			
Understand how a duty of care contributes to safe practice	☐ I know this	☐ Satisfactory	☐ I should review this	☐ This is new to me
Aware of the support available to help address dilemmas arising out of a duty of care	☐ I know this	☐ Satisfactory	☐ I should review this	☐ This is new to me
Understand how to deal with incidents, errors and any near misses	☐ I know this	☐ Satisfactory	☐ I should review this	☐ This is new to me
Highlight the legal and ethical issues associated with a duty	☐ I know this	☐ Satisfactory	☐ I should review this	☐ This is new to me
Discuss the ways in which confrontation and difficult situations can be dealt with	☐ I know this	☐ Satisfactory	☐ I should review this	☐ This is new to me
Describe adverse events, errors and near misses	☐ I know this	☐ Satisfactory	☐ I should review this	☐ This is new to me

Introduction

People who are receiving services provided by health and social care workers should be able to trust those people with regards to their health and wellbeing. In order to justify that trust every health and social care provider has a duty to maintain a good standard of practice and care and to show respect for human life. As a healthcare support worker, you have a professional duty of

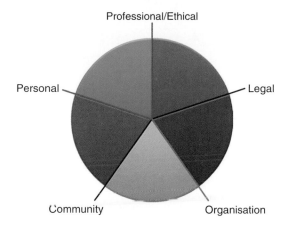

Figure 5.1   Duty of care.

care to the people you provide care and support to. This duty is different to any relationship you may have, for example, with your friends and family.

Those providing care have a responsibility to reduce or limit the amount of harm or injury that may be experienced by the people they offer services to. The principle of duty of care is that those providing care or support to others have an obligation to avoid acts or omissions that could be reasonably foreseen (predicted) to injure or harm other people. This means that those offering care and support must anticipate risks for those being cared for and take care to prevent them from coming to harm (physical and emotional harm).

Duty of care

Duty of care is an expression that is used in many ways. It is often used to describe the obligations that are contained within your role as a health or social care worker. As a health or social care worker you owe a duty of care to your patients, those who use your services, the people you work with, your employer, yourself and the public interest (Figure 5.1). Everyone has a duty of care – this is not something that you can opt out of.

The law insists on a duty of care for all practitioners, all occupations and all levels. This applies regardless of whether you are a healthcare assistant, assistant practitioner, student, registered nurse, doctor or other, whether you are employed full time or part time, or by an agency or in a temporary role, and whether you are a volunteer, registered or non-registered. The practitioner has a legal responsibility for the care they are providing, which applies even if you are not directly responsible for the person's care.

The duty of care is imposed when it is 'reasonably foreseeable' that harm could be caused to patients by staff as a result of their actions or their failure to act (omissions). The duty of care to the people being cared for exists as soon as they are accepted for treatment or a task is accepted and they commence receiving services.

Your duty of care

Your duty of care will mean that you have to aspire to offer high-quality care to the best of your ability, and if there are any reasons why you are unable to do this then you must make this known – you must say so.

Thinking cap 5.1

Duty of care

Make a list of who the law imposes a duty of care on and where and when this exists:

Duty of care imposed on	When it exists

It is expected that you will maintain a reasonable standard of care. You will be required to:

- Keep your knowledge and skills up to date.
- Provide a service that will be of no less a quality than that to be expected based on the skills, responsibilities and the range of activities within your particular trade or profession.
- Be in a position to know what has to be done to make sure that the service you provide is safe.
- Maintain accurate and contemporaneous records of your work.
- Not delegate work nor accept any delegated work, unless it is clear that the person to whom the work is delegated is competent to carry out the work in a safe and appropriately skilled way.
- Safeguard confidential information unless the wider duty of care or the public interest may justify disclosure.

As well as you owing a duty of care, your employer also owes a duty of care. All employees have obligations and rights, and these arise from the contract of employment.

Employers have a duty to provide all staff with clear roles and responsibilities, as well as providing the appropriate training. You should not be asked to perform any task that exceeds your level of competence. If you are being required to take on tasks that you are not properly equipped for or trained to do then you must decline this request explaining why.

Concerns

The notion of duty of care may sometimes seem overwhelming. The responsibility owed to one party (the employer), for example, could conflict with the responsibility to the people being cared for or supported. The duty of care can be seen as a balancing act and there are several aspects that must be given consideration:

- Legal – what does the law suggest?
- Professional/ethical – what do other workers expect?
- Employer – what do our employers say we should do (agreed ways of working)?
- Society – what do society and other members of the community expect?
- Personal – what are our own beliefs and values suggesting?

Agreed ways of working have been discussed in Chapter 3. To react to possible harmful situations you should know how to respond and how to report any concerns. One aspect of your duty

Stop, look, respond 5.1

Balancing act

In Figure 5.1 some of the elements associated with duty of care have been outlined. There are times when conflict can occur; can you think of what some of these might be in the place where you work?

Some examples might include balancing the safety of the person you care for or offer support to against other concerns such as:

- the safety of other people/your personal safety;
- other rights of people who use services, such as the right to privacy;
- the aims of the service, for example, aiming to empower people;
- the amount of information you give to others about those you care for or offer support to.

Discuss two issues or dilemmas where you think conflict could occur:

Issue 1
Issue 2

of care is to pass on any concerns that you have. Concerns might be about anything from poor working conditions or equipment to staff who have been untrained, as well as suspected abuse. If in any situation you do not know what you should do then you must ask your manager. Some of the most common issues that those working in health and social care raise concerns about are related to workloads, staffing and skill mix.

Promoting independence

There will be times when your duty to care (safeguarding the wellbeing of the individual) is in conflict with your duty to promote the individual's right to take risks. You must take note and remember that you have a duty to ensure an individual is kept safe and that the person experiences no harm. However, these situations can raise dilemmas, and there may be times when you might not know what is the right thing to do in order to keep the person safe whilst at the same time assisting them to make choices of their own.

Thinking cap 5.2

Safe staffing levels

If you have good reason to suppose that workloads, skill mix, the working environment or other working arrangements may not be safe, your duty of care requires that you raise your concerns; you must not stay silent.

Think about the ways you might go about raising concerns in your work place.

Stop, look, respond 5.2

Respect

To respect somebody is to show esteem or regard for, or to honour another person.
   What does respect mean to you?
   Do you think that your understanding of respect may differ from the understanding of those people you support or care for?
   What might disrespect look like, feel like for you?

When providing care or offering support there can be occasions when the choices made by people can lead you to think that they are unwise, reckless, or unsafe, and you may disagree with them – for example, when someone decides to continue to engage in unsafe sex, or to have a termination of pregnancy or to eat foods that have a high fat content.

Providing information

People make decisions all the time. However, there are occasions when an individual may not be able to understand and retain the information that is required to make a decision or make known their preferences. They may lack the mental capacity to make the decision, and if this is the case then additional advice or guidance is needed, so as to ensure that the person's choice is respected.

One aspect of your role will be to offer people as much information as possible regarding the choices that they have decided to make and to discuss with them the consequences of their choices (it should be noted that the information provided must be offered in such a way that the person is able to understand and weigh up the issues). Offer information in such a way that the person can make their own decision, even if you consider that their decision involves risk. Undertaking a risk assessment can help to identify if there are any ways in which risks may be reduced and how the individual can be supported when making decisions concerning their health and wellbeing.

The person's health and wellbeing must at all times be your key priority. Always seek advice from your manager if you have any concerns or if you are unsure.

Thinking cap 5.3

Providing information

Think about the ways in which you can offer information to people in order to ensure that they understand the key issues being discussed.

   Think about a variety of media that you could use and also consider the opportunities and challenges that a multi-media approach may bring.

The constitution, complaints, comments and compliments

The NHS Constitution explains the principles and values of the NHS. It is applicable only to England; nevertheless it contains some principles that may apply to other countries within the UK. The constitution sets out rights to which patients, public and staff are entitled as well as outlining the pledges that the NHS is committed to, reinforcing the message that the NHS operates in a fair and effective manner.

By law the Secretary of State for Health, all NHS bodies, private and voluntary sector providers supplying NHS services and local authorities are required to take account of the constitution when making decisions and taking any action.

When someone is unhappy with the services that you provide, it is important to let them know their rights when it comes to making a complaint. These rights are outlined in the NHS constitution when the complaint concerns the NHS.

Raising concerns

An updated NHS constitution has been produced by the Department of Health. Areas that have been changed with the aim of improvement include:

- patient involvement;
- feedback;
- duty of candour;
- end of life care;
- integrated care;
- complaints;
- patient information;
- staff rights, responsibilities and commitments;
- dignity, respect and compassion.

The organisation in which you work has arrangements in place that will allow people to complain if they are dissatisfied with the services they receive. People can if they wish (often when they are unsure whether to make a complaint) discuss the matter with the Patient Liaison Advisory Service (PALS) locally. The Complaints Advocacy Service may also be approached to provide advice.

 Stop, look, respond 5.3

Complaints

Think about your place of work and how the complaints procedure works there. Could you explain how the complaints procedure works to a person you care for or support?

If not, meet with a senior colleague and go through this procedure, noting the various processes associated with it. It is important to understand the various processes as they usually have time restraints and certain things need to be done within set time frames.

When people provide you and your colleagues with positive comments and you receive compliments this can be a really good motivator. This can encourage staff and demonstrate how your ways of working can have a positive impact on people.

Untoward incidents

There are many words and phrases used to describe untoward incidents, such as adverse events, adverse clinical incidents, errors, near misses and incidents (Table 5.1).

Unfortunately, despite having procedures and policies in place, harm does occur to people whom we care for and offer support to. Mistakes happen, for a number of reasons; for example:

- negligence;
- lack of understanding and knowledge;
- ineffective communication;
- excessive workloads;
- stress;
- failure to work as a team.

Stop, look, respond 5.4

Incident forms

Every employer should have in place detailed arrangements for reporting adverse incidents. Do you know what these detailed arrangements are?

Your workplace will have a form that is specifically used for the recording of incidents, accidents and near misses (this is an incident reporting system). On this form you will be asked to record details of the incident, such as the date, time and facts.

Find the form or ask your manager for a copy of it and have a look at the details on it.

Table 5.1   Events, errors, near misses and incidents

Issue	Comment
Adverse event	An event or omission that arises during care provision, causing physical or psychological injury to a person being cared for or being supported. Action or lack of action that leads to unexpected, unintended and preventable harm. An adverse event can be seen as an event that could have caused, or did result in, harm to people or groups of people
Error	The failure to complete a planned action as intended, or the use of an incorrect plan of action to accomplish a given aim. Not doing something as it should have been done, such as bad planning or forgetfulness
Near miss	Situation in which an event or omission, or a sequence of events or omissions, arising during care provision fails to develop further, whether or not as the result of compensating action, preventing injury to a patient. These are situations where an action could have harmed a person but, by chance or purpose, this harm was prevented
Incident	A serious event in which a person or people were harmed or could have been harmed. Serious incidents are described as events that need investigation as they caused severe harm or damage to either the person receiving care or support or the organisation

Negligence

There is a difference between making an allegation of negligence and making a complaint. There is a difference between making a complaint and a clinical negligence claim. Usually the key reason for making a complaint is to get answers about what went wrong. When making a complaint the complainant may also seek an apology or be told that as a result of the complaint there will be changes to practice to help prevent mistakes from occurring again. In a clinical negligence case, the person making the claim is usually seeking money after an injury or death. If anything other than compensation is being sought then consideration should be given to making a formal complaint.

For a claim of negligence to be successful the following elements must be satisfied:

- A duty of care existed.
- There was a breach in the standard of care.
- Reasonably foreseeable harm was caused.
- There was a clear chain of causation between the negligent act and the harm that was caused.

Conflict

Conflict can occur at work or outside of work; conflict is unavoidable when working with others. Team members often have a number of different perspectives, and there are times when those differences could turn into conflict.

Conflict can arise for many reasons, between individuals, groups and teams, such as: a disagreement, differences in values, attitudes, needs, or expectations, miscommunication or insufficient information. Conflict or challenging behaviour can occur as a result of distress or because needs are not being met.

Healthy conflict (constructive conflict) can be good for a team as this can result in positive and constructive challenges as well as bringing about learning; it should be seen as an opportunity for growth. See Table 5.2 for some tips on how to manage conflict.

Responding to conflict

People respond to conflict in many ways, for example:

- Avoidance – results in not addressing the conflict (issues).
- Competition – results in championing one's own goals at the expense of another; this becomes a win-lose situation.

Table 5.2   Some tips on how to manage conflict

- Be aware of tensions before they are able to escalate
- As soon as possible, talk to individuals early, establishing the reason(s) for conflict
- Be open to resolving issues and talk things through; encourage immediate resolution; this may prevent any build-up of tension
- Remain objective; deal with facts as opposed to emotion
- Try not to let conflict become personal
- Establish the facts before making any judgment
- Address conflict in an open way
- Respect and protect any confidential information being discussed
- When people are treated with respect and dignity it can be easier to arrive at a solution

- Accommodation – results in meeting the goals of the other person; a lose-win situation. This approach might be appropriate when the issue or goal is more important than winning, the other individual is more powerful, or when an individual is wrong.
- Compromise – combines assertiveness and cooperation; a lose-lose situation.
- Collaboration – results in finding a mutually agreeable solution; a win-win situation.

When two or more people view things or situations from different perspectives, then these relationships can be compromised by conflict. Conflict when managed effectively can lead to personal and organisational growth. If it is not managed effectively, this can impact on a health or social care worker's ability to provide quality care and support.

Chapter summary

- Duty of care is a legal requirement, applying as soon as someone receives care or treatment. Failing to adhere to this duty can result in legal action.
- The duty of care applies to all staff; staff cannot choose whether or not to accept a duty of care. The duty of care applies to other people you work with.
- There are procedures in place that will enable you to raise concerns regarding issues associated with duty of care.
- In order to promote independence you are required to work in such a way that you respect and protect the person's rights; this includes their right to make their own choices and to take risks.
- Providing people with information in a way and in a format they can use can help with regards to their decision-making.
- There are times when people wish to make a complaint about the service provided. You have a duty to ensure that people are aware that they have a right to complain or comment about their care or support.
- People also make compliments about service provision and this can help to motivate and encourage staff.
- Despite working in such a way as to prevent harm and enhance health and wellbeing there are times when mistakes do happen. There are a number of reasons these mistakes happen.
- Conflict can occur at work or outside of work; it is unavoidable when working with others. Understanding why conflict can occur can help to manage this inevitable aspect of working.

 Case scenario 5.1

Janice

Janice is 42 years old; both her mother and her one sister have been diagnosed with breast cancer; Janice has been called for a breast screen; Janice has a learning disability. The support worker providing support to Janice has used a range of media to explain to Janice what this test is about and what options she has. She has explained the consequences of not having the test.

Janice has decided that she does not want the breast screen and that she thinks the test is rude. The manager of the residential service where Janice lives is insistent that she goes for the test despite Janice's protestations, as the manager thinks the test is in Janice's best interests.

Janice has an advocate and she is engaged to ensure that Janice's voice is heard. At a care planning meeting it is decided that Janice has the right to refuse this screen despite the manager's unhappiness.

Are there any other options available that may help Janice to make an informed decision?

Resource file

UNISON
Duty of care handbook
https://www.unison.org.uk/content/uploads/2013/06/On-line-Catalogue197863.pdf

Public Concern at Work: The Whistleblowing Charity
http://www.pcaw.org.uk

Chapter 6

Equality and diversity

Care certificate outcomes

1. Understand the importance of equality and inclusion.
2. Work in an inclusive way.
3. Access information, advice and support about diversity, equality and inclusion.

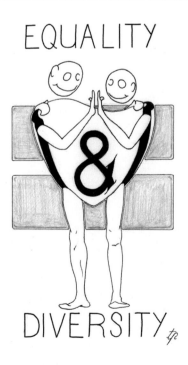

Fundamentals of Care: A Textbook for Health and Social Care Assistants, First Edition. Ian Peate.
© 2017 John Wiley & Sons Ltd. Published 2017 by John Wiley & Sons Ltd.

Take stock

Rate your current knowledge and skills prior to reading this chapter. Put a tick in the box that you think applies to you with regards to the standard being discussed:

Key:
I know this I have a good level of knowledge or skills regarding this aspect of the standard. I make use of the knowledge and skills identified on a regular basis, feeling confident in my ability and performance. I do not need a refresher.
Satisfactory My level of knowledge and standard of skills meet the criteria associated with the standard. I use the skills and knowledge from time to time. I might not always feel confident in my capability. I would benefit from a refresher.
I require a review I do not feel that I have the skills and/or the knowledge that would enable me to meet the standard in a confident and competent way. The knowledge and skills I used to have are no longer valid. I will require a refresher.
This is new to me I have never worked in a caring role before or I have never covered this topic before. I will need further training and development in this area.

Standard	Self-assessment			
Understand the terms equality and diversity	☐ I know this	☐ Satisfactory	☐ I should review this	☐ This is new to me
Discuss the ways in which you can work in an inclusive way	☐ I know this	☐ Satisfactory	☐ I should review this	☐ This is new to me
Able to reflect on diversity in the health and social care setting concerning gender, ethnicity, disability, religion, sexuality, class and age	☐ I know this	☐ Satisfactory	☐ I should review this	☐ This is new to me
Highlight aspects associated with inequality in health and social care	☐ I know this	☐ Satisfactory	☐ I should review this	☐ This is new to me
Understand the impact of labelling, stereotyping and prejudice	☐ I know this	☐ Satisfactory	☐ I should review this	☐ This is new to me
Demonstrate cultural sensitivity	☐ I know this	☐ Satisfactory	☐ I should review this	☐ This is new to me

Introduction

Equality and diversity are becoming important in all aspects of our lives including whilst we are at work. We are living in an increasingly diverse society, and because of this there is a need to be able to respond appropriately and sensitively to this diversity.

When equality and diversity become a part of all aspects of how we work this will ensure that the people we work with and our colleagues are valued, motivated and treated fairly. Working in this way demonstrates that you are able to meet the needs of everyone. In order to work in a non-discriminatory manner you have to understand what the key issues and the key terms mean and incorporate them into your work.

A care provider who provides services to meet the diverse needs of those who use those services is likely to find that delivering its core business in this way will be more efficient. Furthermore, a workforce that has a supportive working environment in which to work will be more productive.

Legislation

There are many aspects of the health and care worker's role that are governed by law (some elements of legislation are outlined in Table 6.1). Every person in the UK has rights and freedoms irrespective of their situation or characteristics. Equality and inclusion can be seen as basic human rights.

Equality duty

The Equality Act 2010 came into force in October 2010, providing a modern, single legal framework with clear, streamlined law to more effectively tackle disadvantage and discrimination.

The Act simplifies, strengthens and harmonises the current legislation to provide a discrimination law that aims to protect individuals from unfair treatment and promotes a fair and more equal society. The nine main pieces of legislation that have merged are identified in Table 6.2.

Table 6.1   Some elements of legislation that impact on the role and function of the health and care worker

Legislation	Discussion
The Human Rights Act 1998	Describes the way that everyone should be treated by the state and by public authorities
The Mental Capacity Act 2005	Provided to protect people who are unable to make decisions for themselves
The Equality Act 2010	Came into force in October 2010 providing a modern, single legal framework with a clear, streamlined law to tackle disadvantage and discrimination
The Health and Social Care Act 2012	This Act aims to modernise NHS care by supporting new services and providing people with a greater voice in their care
The Care Act 2014	At the heart of this Act is the principle of wellbeing aiming to bring care and support legislation together. It aims to make care and support clearer and fairer and to put the wellbeing of people at the centre of decisions and to include and develop further personalisation

Table 6.2   The nine main pieces of legislation that have merged to become the Equality Act 2010

1. The Equal Pay Act 1970
2. The Sex Discrimination Act 1975
3. The Race Relations Act 1976
4. The Disability Discrimination Act 1995
5. The Employment Equality (Religion or Belief) Regulations 2003
6. The Employment Equality (Sexual Orientation) Regulations 2003
7. The Employment Equality (Age) Regulations 2006
8. The Equality Act 2006, Part 2
9. The Equality Act (Sexual Orientation) Regulations 2007

Table 6.3   Protected characteristics

- Age
- Disability
- Gender reassignment
- Pregnancy and maternity
- Race (including ethnic or national origins, colour or nationality)
- Religion or belief (including lack of belief)
- Sex
- Sexual orientation
- Marriage and civil partnership

The Act requires any public organisation (e.g. councils, hospitals, police, schools, government departments, fire and transport authorities) to think about how they can make sure their work supports equality. For example, in the services they provide, through their jobs and through the money they spend. This is in addition to their duty not to discriminate.

When public authorities perform their functions, the Equality Act says that they must have due regard or consider the need to:

1. Eliminate unlawful discrimination.
2. Advance equality of opportunity between people who share a protected characteristic (see Table 6.3) and those who do not.
3. Foster or encourage good relations between those who share a protected characteristic and those who do not.

Having due regard requires public authorities to consciously consider or think about the need to do the three things set out in the public sector equality duty. It is the courts that will make the decision to determine if a public authority has done enough to conform to the duty.

Human Rights Act

Human rights are rights and freedoms that are based on the core assumption that everyone is entitled to dignity, equality and respect. The Human Rights Act 1998 is composed of a series of sections that have the effect of organising the protections in the European Convention on Human Rights into UK law.

All public bodies (e.g. courts, police, local governments, hospitals, publicly funded schools) and other bodies carrying out public functions have to comply with the Convention's rights.

The Act sets out the fundamental rights and freedoms that individuals in the UK have access to. They include:

- Right to life.
- Freedom from torture and inhumane or degrading treatment.
- Right to liberty and security.
- Right to a fair trial.
- No punishment without law.
- Respect for your private and family life, home and correspondence.
- Freedom of thought, belief and religion.
- Freedom of expression.
- Freedom of assembly and association.

- Right to marry and start a family.
- Protection from discrimination in respect of these rights and freedoms.
- Right to a peaceful enjoyment of your property.
- Right to education.
- Right to participate in free elections.

Defining terms

Definitions are open to debate, and you may hear different views of what constitutes equality. Often the terms equality and diversity are used interchangeably; however, the two terms are not the same.

Equality

This is concerned with providing everyone with the opportunity to participate in order to fulfil their potential; it aims to produce a fairer society and is about creating a level playing field. Equality is about treating people alike in response to their needs; people should be given equality of opportunity. You may need, for example, to provide information to people in different formats, consider using assistive technology, such as using Makaton, provide a document in large type or ensure that there are clear and unambiguous signs to departments and buildings for accessibility.

By eliminating prejudice and discrimination, the NHS can deliver services that are personal, fair and diverse and a society that is healthier and happier. An equalities approach appreciates that who we are – based on social categories such as gender, ethnicity, disability, age, social class, sexuality and religion – does not impact on our life experiences, health and wellbeing.

Diversity

Diversity equates to difference; it is about recognising individual and also group differences, acknowledging people as individuals, and placing positive value on diversity in the community and in the workforce. A one-size-fits-all approach is unacceptable. All of us are different; what makes a person unique are the many different parts of that person's character and their identity.

Individual and group diversity must be given consideration in order to ensure that everybody's needs are understood and responded to in effective and respectful ways.

Inclusion

Inclusion is closely associated with diversity and equality, and is about being included within either a group or society as a whole. Whilst it is important to understand the differences in people and in so doing include them and treat them equally and fairly, it must be remembered that people can feel excluded if they are not given an opportunity to take part in group or wider societal activities.

A holistic approach means concerning the whole person taking into account physical, social, economic, psychological, spiritual and other factors, making a commitment to and recognition of inclusivity, equality and diversity. When people are excluded based on their differences, then this is known as discrimination.

Discrimination

Discrimination is an action that is often founded on a person's negative attitude towards others. It is the unjust or prejudicial treatment of different categories of people, for example, on the grounds of ethnicity, ability, age or gender.

Discrimination occurs when one person makes a judgement about another person because of what they are: it could be their appearance, or gender, or religion or any other aspect of their background – for example, assuming that a man is not sensitive enough for a nursing job, or assuming that someone without qualifications lacks intelligence.

Discrimination refers to less favourable treatment because of a person's protected characteristics. Discrimination is prejudices put into action.

Stop, look, respond 6.1

Defining terms

Provide a definition of the following terms and some examples related to your work:

Term	Definition	Example
Equality		
Diversity		
Inclusion		
Discrimination		

The first step in addressing discrimination is to acknowledge the problem; it is everybody's responsibility. It is unacceptable for anyone to experience discrimination, and it should be challenged whenever it is found, be this in your own work, or in the work of others – discrimination is illegal. Working in a reflective way can help you to identify if and where your own values and beliefs are leading to discriminating treatment of others. If you are aware that individuals are being treated unfairly, you should discuss this with your manager, who will then take action to ensure that the poor practice is challenged in an appropriate way and to encourage positive change.

In order to prevent discrimination the health and social care worker should:

- Be positive about an individual's life history, their family and friends.
- Encourage independence after risk has been assessed.
- Recognise an individual as a person of worth.
- Do not judge or stereotype an individual.
- Do not make unfair judgments about an individual because of your own attitude.

Labelling, stereotyping and prejudice

Labelling, stereotyping and prejudice can lead to discrimination. When people are discriminated against they are treated differently because of the assumptions that are being made about them as an individual or as a group of people based on their differences. When society (individuals in society or society as a whole) exhibits negative attitudes and behaviours then this can lead to individuals or groups being oppressed or disadvantaged and inequality then occurs.

From the moment we begin to learn, we are taught to classify, to sort objects and place them in groups. Whilst this may be fine for objects, this is not acceptable for people. When people are grouped, this is called stereotyping.

Often when we think of images such as man/woman, old/young, gay/straight, hooligan/law abiding, disabled/non-disabled this produces certain mental images. These images may not be based on our own experiences; however, they may be based on a series of misconceptions that we have amassed during our lifetime. Stereotypes can be harmful when we make assumptions about people that are based on their protected characteristic, as opposed to treating them as individuals.

A stereotype may contain some truths about a group, but it must not be assumed to be true of each individual. Messages we get from education, family members and the media all affect the strength of the stereotype.

Prejudice can influence the decisions that we make on a daily basis, leading to the development of discriminatory attitudes about certain people, producing negative views about different lifestyles, value systems, standards of behaviour and the value that is placed on other people's right to choose to be different.

 ## Thinking cap 6.1

Labelling, stereotyping and prejudice

Consider ways in which labelling, stereotyping and prejudice occur and write some notes about this:

Labelling	Stereotyping	Prejudice

 ## Thinking cap 6.2

Prejudice

Identify a time when, on reflection, you had already made up your mind about a person or group of people before you had even met them. You may have decided what they were like based on what another person had told you about them. What effect did that have on your subsequent experience of that person or that group?

Inequality

Care and support should be arranged around individuals, their families, carers and communities. In order to do this effectively those providing care and support must recognise differences and individuality to reduce inequality in health and social care outcomes.

Health and social care inequalities are differences in health and social status driven by inequalities in society. Health is shaped by a number of different factors, for example lifestyle, wealth, educational achievement, availability of work, job security, housing conditions, geographical location, psycho-social stress and discrimination. Health inequalities represent the increasing effect of these factors over a person's lifetime; they can be passed on from one generation to the next in a number of ways, for example, through maternal influences on baby and child development.

All health and support care workers must work in a holistic, non-judgmental, caring and sensitive way that avoids assumptions, supports social inclusion, acknowledges and values individual choice, and recognises diversity. Where needed, they should challenge inequality, discrimination and exclusion from access to care.

Stop, look, respond 6.2

Health and social care inequality

Health and social inequality refers to gaps in the quality of health and social healthcare across racial, ethnic, gender, sexual orientation and socio-economic groups. Geographical location, employment status and income are also known to be important influences in shaping an individual's ability to access health and social care and in experiencing positive health and social care outcomes.

In the table below consider the groups identified as at risk and then think about ways in which the issues described can be addressed.

Groups at risk	Notes on addressing factors
Socio-economically disadvantaged communities Risk factors for poor health are more prevalent among those populations who are deprived populations; these include smoking, obesity, lack of physical exercise, high blood pressure, poor and congested housing, unemployment, poor educational attainment, low income, residence in inner cities, exposure to crime and violence.	
People with disabilities Living with illness and impairment makes economic hardship much harder to avoid. Continuing health difficulties and the discrimination with which they are associated can increase the risk of unemployment, dependency on welfare benefits and long-term poverty.	
Black, Asian and minority ethnic communities Those men born in South Asia but now resident in England are 50% more likely to have a heart attack or angina than men in the general population. Immigrants from Bangladesh have the highest rates, followed by Pakistanis, then Indians and other South Asians. Men born in the Caribbean and now living in England by contrast are 50% more likely to die of stroke than the general population but they have much lower mortality from coronary heart disease.	
Asylum seekers/refugees Formal barriers (e.g. legislation) reduce access to services for those people who have recently arrived, in particular refugees and asylum seekers. Ninety-five per cent of asylum seekers in London have been refused GP registration at least once in the preceding 12 months. This issue is made worse by a lack of knowledge (on the part of both service providers and service users) about legal entitlements to public services.	

People with learning disabilities and those with mental health problems

People with learning disabilities and people with mental health problems are much more likely than other people to have significant health risks and major health problems. Health problems for people with learning disabilities include, for example, obesity and respiratory disease; those with mental health problems include obesity, smoking, heart disease, high blood pressure, respiratory disease, diabetes and stroke. Both of these groups are likely to die younger than other people.

The government is working to put in place processes that will reduce these inequalities, for instance by encouraging access to primary care services such as the promotion of screening programmes with the GP, training health and social care workers to pay particular attention to the needs of these groups, national targeting of these groups and raising awareness of their needs, and monitoring progress.

Cultural sensitivity

Culture is a complex concept and can be considered to include the learning, sharing and communication of values, beliefs, norms and ways of life of a specific group that directs their thinking, the ways in which they make decisions and the actions that they take. Health and social care workers are required to take into account the diversity of the social and cultural worlds inhabited by the people they provide care to or offer support to.

Cultural belief systems interact with all aspects of information processing. A culturally competent health and social care provider must develop cultural sensitivity.

Thinking cap 6.3

Culture

Within your local health or social care setting identify the diverse groups that are currently in receipt of health and/or social care. Think about those people whose first language is not English. How would you go about ensuring that their diverse needs are met?

Cultural sensitivity for those who work in health and social care can be seen as sensitivity to the ways in which people's values and perceptions about healthcare can and often do differ from those who offer care or provide support. As populations continually grow and the percentage of minorities steadily increases, cultural sensitivity is a key element of the care and support the health or social care worker provides, improving the continuity of care and patient satisfaction.

Thinking cap 6.4

Resources

Identify/compile a list of resources available to help meet the specific needs of the local population that you serve. What are they? Are they readily available? What could be improved?

A person's culture and ethnicity will determine how they perceive the world. Growth and development in a particular environment will set the stage for those values and beliefs a person will have throughout his or her life. These different environments provide a person with a unique 'web' – webs of significance whereby each person has their own web in which the everyday lives of people are rooted. Within this web there are reasons why people understand the world differently and assign meaning to events and ideas that others would not. The web adds to who people are as individuals. It not only consists of having a particular eye colour, a certain type of hair and colour of skin, it also includes experiences, for example, being supported, comforted and feeling safe.

People carry with them cultures and customs that will affect the ways in which they interpret the world, their experiences and their relationships. These also include how they interpret their health and social care provision, their experiences of health and social care, and the relationships they may have had with health and social care providers. When people face crises, or they lose control over aspects of their life due to illness, then their core beliefs and value systems are more likely to be held more strongly.

Behaviours that are usually associated with response to disability and illness, for example fear, pain, and anxiety, are culturally determined.

Thinking cap 6.5

Interacting

Reflect on an interaction with a person you offer care to or provide support to that was frustrated by culture, language, disability, gender, age, religion or belief, sexual orientation or other. How could this interaction have been improved?

Stop, look, respond 6.3

Cultural affiliations

Within the area where you work identify a person to whom you provide care or offer support who is from a cultural background that differs from yours. Provide an example of how your understanding of a different culture and value system helps you to address health and social care needs, ensuring that the person is at the centre of all that is done.

Use the following table to organise your thinking; you can also make a comparison between yourself and the person chosen.

Characteristic	Person identified	Self
Age		
Gender		
Religion		
Family		

Characteristic	Person identified	Self
Cultural heritage		
Language		
Nationality		
Community		
Other _____		
Other _____		
Other _____		

Thinking cap 6.6

Questions to consider

1. What inequalities exist?
2. Who is disadvantaged and in what way?
3. What activities is your place of work undertaking to reduce and/or eliminate these inequalities?
4. How can you improve the way you work in order to ensure that you do not make existing health inequalities worse?

Chapter summary

- We all have a responsibility for the quality of the health and social care we provide.
- It is important to ensure that equality of access is at the heart of care and support, and all staff should be able to demonstrate this.
- Every person, whatever their background, should expect to receive the same standard of care from health and social services.
- Equal societies protect and promote equality, real freedom and opportunity to live in the way people value and would choose; in this way everyone can flourish.
- An equal society recognises that people have different needs, situations and goals, removing barriers that limit what people can do and can be.
- There is much legislation concerning equality. In the UK everyone has rights and freedoms irrespective of their situation or characteristics.
- Discrimination happens when one person makes a decision about another because of what they are; this could be based on appearance, gender, religion or any other aspect of their background.
- Labelling, stereotyping and prejudice can lead to discrimination.

Health and social care workers must take into account the social and cultural worlds inhabited by the people they provide care to or offer support to.

Case scenario 6.1

Waadi and Sean

Waadi is a Muslim student and has asked for some flexibility in the school timetable in order to fit in with his religious commitments that are linked to the month of Ramadan. He has requested not to have to take part in physical education classes that are held in the afternoons during the month of Ramadan, since at this time Waadi will be fasting. His request has been denied and he is being required to attend PE classes in the afternoon.

   Another boy, Sean, has requested some flexibility in the timetable for him to fit in with his confirmation classes at his church. Sean is granted permission to leave class half an hour early on Fridays.

Is this discriminatory activity towards Waadi? What type of discrimination? On what grounds is this discrimination?

Resource file

British Institute of Human Rights
An organisation providing people with authoritative and accessible information regarding human rights.
https://www.bihr.org.uk

Stonewall
A lesbian, gay, bisexual and transgender rights charity.
http://www.stonewall.org.uk

The Equality Trust
The Equality Trust works to improve the quality of life in the UK by reducing economic inequality.
https://www.equalitytrust.org.uk/resources

Chapter 7

Working in a person-centred way

Care certificate outcomes

1. Understand person-centred values.
2. Understand working in a person-centred way.
3. Demonstrate awareness of the individual's immediate environment and make changes to address factors that may be causing discomfort or distress.
4. Make others aware of any actions they may be undertaking that are causing discomfort or distress to individuals.
5. Support individuals to minimise pain or discomfort.
6. Support the individual to maintain their identity and self-esteem.
7. Support the individual using person-centred values.

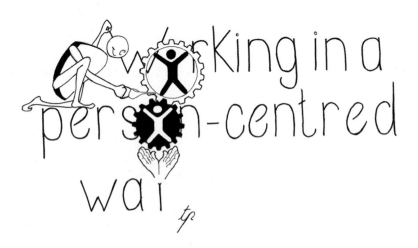

Fundamentals of Care: A Textbook for Health and Social Care Assistants, First Edition. Ian Peate.
© 2017 John Wiley & Sons Ltd. Published 2017 by John Wiley & Sons Ltd.

Take stock

Rate your current knowledge and skills prior to reading this chapter. Put a tick in the box that you think applies to you with regards to the standard being discussed:

Key:
I know this I have a good level of knowledge or skills regarding this aspect of the standard. I make use of the knowledge and skills identified on a regular basis, feeling confident in my ability and performance. I do not need a refresher.
Satisfactory My level of knowledge and standard of skills meet the criteria associated with the standard. I use the skills and knowledge from time to time. I might not always feel confident in my capability. I would benefit from a refresher.
I require a review I do not feel that I have the skills and/or the knowledge that would enable me to meet the standard in a confident and competent way. The knowledge and skills I used to have are no longer valid. I will require a refresher.
This is new to me I have never worked in a caring role before or I have never covered this topic before. I will need further training and development in this area.

Standard	Self-assessment			
Understand person-centred values	☐ I know this	☐ Satisfactory	☐ I should review this	☐ This is new to me
Discuss the ways in which person-centred care and support can be offered	☐ I know this	☐ Satisfactory	☐ I should review this	☐ This is new to me
Consider how values can have a positive and negative impact on how we think and react	☐ I know this	☐ Satisfactory	☐ I should review this	☐ This is new to me
Describe and discuss the 6Cs	☐ I know this	☐ Satisfactory	☐ I should review this	☐ This is new to me
Understand and appreciate the changing needs of the individual	☐ I know this	☐ Satisfactory	☐ I should review this	☐ This is new to me
Highlight the need to support people in order to maintain their identity and self-esteem	☐ I know this	☐ Satisfactory	☐ I should review this	☐ This is new to me

Introduction

The challenges that face the NHS, the independent and voluntary sectors are well understood. In the UK there are growing numbers of older people and people who are living with long-term conditions and disabilities. In order to provide high-quality care that offers people the best possible quality of life, the relationship between people and the services that are provided needs to be given much consideration.

In person-centred care, health and social care professionals work together with the people who use the services. Person-centred care provides support to people with the intention of developing their knowledge, skills and confidence to manage more effectively and to enable them to make informed decisions concerning their own health and healthcare. It is provided in such a way that it reflects the needs of the individual. Most importantly person-centredness ensures that people are always treated with dignity, compassion and respect.

Working in a person-centred way

The positive and negative impact of values (our own and those of the people we provide care to or support) has already been mentioned in previous chapters. Everyday we all of us live our lives according to a set of values; these influence how we think and react. Values are beliefs and ideas about how people should behave; they are shaped very much by our childhoods (upbringing), families, backgrounds, cultures, religions and relationships. These values interrelate and impact on our lives (Figure 7.1).

It is acknowledged that we all have our own values; there are also values that inform the way we are expected to work in health and social care. Some of these work values may reflect our own values, but it may also be the case that our personal values conflict with our work values.

Engaging in a person-centred way where the person is at the centre of all that is done, means that care and support provision must fit the individual, as opposed to the individual being made to fit existing routines or ways of doing things (this is also known as 'one size fits all'). This is key to person-centred working. When the health or social worker adopts person-centred values then they are working in a person-centred way. This requires empowering people to make choices about how their needs are to be met when they may be unable to meet them for themselves (Table 7.1). Empowering a person means to give them the confidence, voice and power for them to speak out on their own behalf and for them to feel that they are in control of their actions.

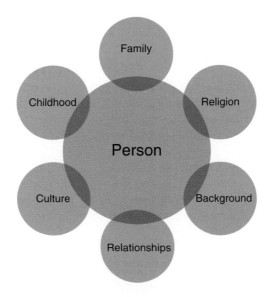

Figure 7.1   The interrelationship of values and the person.

Table 7.1 Working in a person-centred way

- People must be respected as individuals; strive to help them to preserve their dignity at all times
- Engage with the person or their family or carers within their cultural environments in a way that is accepting and anti-discriminatory, free from harassment and exploitation
- Work with people in a warm, sensitive and compassionate way
- Engage in a therapeutic manner and actively listen to their needs and concerns; respond in such a way that responses are helpful; offer information that is clear, accurate, meaningful and jargon free
- Protect and keep confidential all information relating to the person
- Gain the person's consent that is firmly based on a sound understanding and informed choice before any intervention, ensuring that their rights in decision-making and consent will be valued and maintained

The needs of the people and the communities that health and care workers serve must be at the heart of all that is done. Responding to the individual needs and respecting individual choices can help to demonstrate that the needs of the people and, if appropriate, their families are being respected. Failing to take choice into account is disrespect.

Thinking cap 7.1

Respect

Can you think of a time (at work or in a social setting) when you have felt disrespect? What made you feel like this? Did you do anything about this? If so what and if not why not?

There is no agreed definition of what is meant by person-centredness. Any definition would only limit the various possibilities of this complex and dynamic entity. Person-centred support is about valuing and respecting the person who is being cared for or supported. When working in a person-centred way this has the potential to lead to a higher level of engagement.

Stop, look, respond 7.1

Person-centredness

Reflect on the sort of care you would like to receive should you need to be cared for or supported.

> I want those people who care for me to:
> -
> -
> -
> -
> -
> -
> -
> -

(Continued)

Did your responses include any of the following:
   I want those people who care for me to:

- Ask me how it is that I want to be cared for
- Listen to me
- Be polite to me and my family
- Be assured that they do not embarrass me
- Help me stay as independent as is possible
- Let me do as much as I safely can for myself
- Leave me to be alone when I want that
- Only share what they know about me with those who need to know

Person-centred values

Person-centred values are the principles that guide and help us to ensure that the interests of the individual receiving care or support will be the centre of everything we do. For example:

- championing individuality;
- promoting independence;
- providing privacy;
- working in partnership;
- offering choice;
- ensuring dignity;
- respecting people;
- upholding rights.

Table 7.2 outlines the various principles.
   The Health Foundation provides a framework made up of four principles denoting person-centred care (Table 7.3).

Table 7.2   The principles associated with person-centred values

Principle	Discussion
Individuality	Each person has their own identity, which includes the colour of their eyes, their skin, their hair, their likes and dislikes, their wishes, desires, needs, values, beliefs and choices
Independence	Supporting a person's independence requires consideration of what they can do for themselves and to empower them to do as much for themselves as possible. Promoting independence does not mean leaving someone to manage by themselves; it is more about agreeing with that person the support they want and require
Privacy	All people should be able to enjoy privacy; they should be provided with a private space and also time to enjoy it when they say they need it When care and support is offered, particularly when this is associated with a person's personal hygiene or when undertaking intimate procedures, then privacy is paramount Privacy is also associated with a person's private information and includes not talking to others about that person's information unless you have been given permission. Even this should only be on a need-to-know basis, with the intention of facilitating an improvement in that person's care and support
Partnership	When the individual and their family are involved in their care and when you work together with others then this is a working partnership. Effective partnership work is enhanced by effective and open communication, trust, valuing and respecting what others say

Table 7.2 (Continued)

Principle	Discussion
Choice	People should be supported to make choices regarding their care and support and be provided with information that they can understand in order for them to make informed choices, regardless if you think the choice being made would not be the choice that you would make
Dignity	Treating a person with respect, acknowledging and valuing their individuality and their beliefs, is to treat a person in a dignified way. For you to provide care in a dignified manner then you must have an open and positive approach. You will have to take time to do things the way the person wants; you must not make assumptions about what it is they want and how it is they want to be treated
Respect	When you respect a person this requires that you show that the person has significance, they are valued as an individual. It means that you appreciate that they have their own ideas, opinions and feelings; even if you might not agree with them, you still respect them
Rights	People have the right to be protected from harm, the right to respect, dignity and equality. These rights are enshrined in law and in the UK it is the Human Rights Act that is the key legislation in this regard

Table 7.3 Health Foundation's four principles that underpin person-centredness

1. Providing people dignity, compassion and respect
2. Ensuring coordinated care, support or treatment
3. Offering personalised care, support or treatment
4. Assisting people to recognise and develop their own strengths and abilities to empower them to live an independent and fulfilling life

 Stop, look, respond 7.2

The 6Cs

Not one of the 6Cs is more important than the other five; each one (the values and behaviours) carries equal weight. The 6Cs focus on ensuring that the person is at the heart of the care they receive. In this table the 6Cs are described. Now you can add in the final column the ways in which you enact the 6Cs as you offer care or provide support.

Component	Definition	Ways in which you enact the 6Cs when caring or supporting others
Care	Having someone's best interests at heart, doing what you can to maintain or improve their wellbeing	
Compassion	Being able to feel for someone, understanding them and their situation	
Competence	To understand what someone needs and have the knowledge and skills to provide it	
Communication	To listen carefully as well as being able to speak and act in a way that the person understands	
Courage	Not to have fear to try out new things or to say if you are concerned about anything	
Commitment	Dedication to providing care and support as well as understanding the responsibility you have as a worker	

Regardless of the specific care or interventions that a person receives, the principles in Table 7.3 should be taken into account. Any aspect of person-centred care, in any health or social care setting, will comprise a mix of these principles.

When a person is highly dependent, for example, if they are unconscious or if they otherwise lack capacity, then there is likely to be more emphasis on some principles than others. It is usually possible to practise all four principles to some extent with all people.

Thinking cap 7.2

The principles

Think about a person you have cared for or offered support to recently. Now with that person in mind think about the principles outlined in Table 7.3 and think about what principles applied in that instance.

Enabling

Generally enablement (a poorly defined term) describes the level to which people feel they are being supported to develop their own unique range of capabilities. There is often overlap with other commonly used terms, for example, activation, health literacy, involvement and participation. The principle of acting in an enabling way is somewhat different from the other terms. Being unique means each person has their own needs that differ from those of others.

For care to be enabling, then the relationship between those who care or offer support to others, and the recipients of that care, has to be one of a partnership. This requires a change in the usual relationship where the care worker is often seen as the expert and the person receiving care simply follows their instructions. It is a relationship in which healthcare workers and those persons receiving care or support work together to appreciate what is important to the person, working together to help make decisions about the person's care and treatment, and to identify and achieve the individual's goals.

We all have a role to play in supporting the people to whom we offer care with the aim of developing their knowledge; skills and confidence are required to fully participate in this partnership. This is also true for healthcare workers, who may have to work in different ways if care is to be enabling.

Coordinated care

Services provided to people should be seamless; this means they should be offered services in a coordinated way; coordinated services should provide support or treatment across multiple episodes and over periods of time. An identified individual should be responsible for coordinating the person's care, support or treatment regardless of where the care episodes take place.

Care coordination becomes critical during the time of transitions between services. In public services transitions occur all the time; for example, a referral from a social worker to a specialist service is seen as a transition. When this occurs the person should be supported in order to make informed decisions, for example about whether or not they wish to see a specialist. This is very different from being 'referred'.

Personalised care

Personalised care focuses on the person, as a person and not as a diagnosis or a set of symptoms. Here the emphasis is about heeding what matters to the person and their family during interactions with those who offer care and support. What it is that matters to the person will depend on the context, where the interactions are taking place and with whom the person is interacting. The person should always be offered care that is tailored to their needs, that is to say personalised care, support or treatment.

Involving the person in a shared decision-making conversation, for example, concerning an impending operation, demonstrates personalisation. Asking the person about their preferences in terms of risks and providing them with information about what is known about specified outcomes concerning the operation from a clinical perspective helps with regards to shared decision-making.

Person-centred planning

A care plan sets out in detail the way daily care and support must be provided to an individual. Care plans are also known as plans of support and individual plans.

A plan of care is one way of supporting those with long-term conditions and disabilities to work together with health and social care professionals to plan their care. This process involves exploring what matters to that person, identifying the best treatment, care and support, and supporting them to set goals and to think about activities that they could take to reach them.

Key elements associated with effective care planning include:

- Engaging people in decisions about their treatment and care and to be able to act on these decisions.
- Being committed to working in partnership with people.
- Having systems in place to organise resources effectively.

Each of the elements is important along with the interdependence of each element; if one element is weak or absent, then the structure is not fit for purpose.

It is important to find out the history, preferences, wishes and needs of the individual if you are to provide care and support that respects that person's wishes, needs and preferences. Depending on where you work it may be you who is required to find out what you can about them. When you take time to find out about their personal history, having a genuine interest in them by talking with them or gathering information about them will give you a deeper insight into who they are as an individual along with their likes and dislikes. When you have this information the care plan can be put together, working with the individual concerned.

Care plans are key sources of information; they are dynamic records that are continually reviewed and updated as a person's needs and preferences change. A review or an evaluation of a care plan considers what is working, what does not work and what may need to change. This is done with the person the care plan had been written for. If a person is unable to swallow as a result of a stroke, for example, then that person's diet will need to change; however, it should still take into account the things they would like to eat and drink. Care plans can also be considered legal documents, and they may be called up to provide evidence if an untoward incident has occurred or a person wishes to make a complaint.

Stop, look, respond 7.3

Care plans

There are different types of care plans. Make sure you understand how they are used where you work. Seek advice from your manager, who will be able to explain how the care plans should be used.

Care plans should be written in such a way that they become a prescription of care. This will enable those who change shift to have current, up-to-date information regarding the individual, allowing them to offer the best possible care that is person-centred. If you think that the care plan of a person with whom you are working needs to be amended or adjusted then you should speak with your manager about this.

Supporting people

An important consideration with regards to person-centred care is that people have an inner desire to fulfil their personal potential. To do this the person must feel safe, and those providing care or support must be non-judgmental and compassionate. Acting in a non-judgmental way requires you to accept the individual for who they are, seeing them as positive and capable of making their own decisions and choices, regardless of what you think. When the person feels safe and they are not being judged then the individual can start to think about what it is that is important to them and make the best decisions.

Person-centred care can be used to improve any aspect of a person's health and wellbeing including, for example, making decisions about end-of-life care, agreeing a treatment plan for a person with ongoing mental health problems, or working with the person during a period of wellness to plan for how their care should look when they are less able to make choices.

When helping people plan to ensure that their needs are met, be these long-term or short-term needs, the aim should be to ensure their future wellbeing and quality of life is improved. Wellbeing is related to those areas identified in Figure 7.2.

Advanced care planning

Taking time to talk to people about their needs is important: ask them what they want as well as what they do not want. It is also essential to note that people can change their minds about things when they want to, and this should be encouraged. In end-of-life-care this is particularly true where a person may not be able to voice their wishes as they may have done before. The person may have planned ahead and expressed what they would like to happen regarding their care if they are unable to decide for themselves anymore. This is known as advanced care.

Different ways of communicating may be needed in these circumstances, for example, involving the work of an advocate who is able to express the person's wishes on their behalf if the person is unable to communicate the information for him or herself. An advocate aims to ensure that people, in particular those in society who are most vulnerable, are able to have their voice heard on issues that are important to them, protect and defend their rights, and ensure that their views and wishes are fully considered when decisions are being made about their lives.

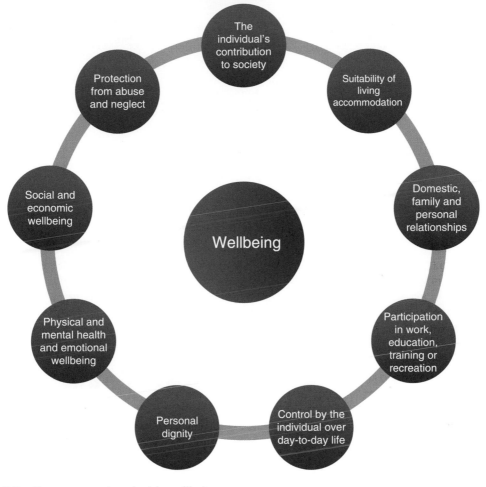

Figure 7.2 Factors associated with wellbeing.

The environment of care

The environment in which people are being cared for can impact either positively or negatively on their health and wellbeing. A person should feel comfortable where they are; this can promote wellbeing. These are some examples of things in the area or the environment around an individual that may cause them discomfort or distress:

- temperature of the room;
- lighting;
- noise;
- unpleasant smells;
- number of people present;
- cleanliness of the environment.

The health or care worker can help to address these issues. Ask the person if there are any environmental issues that they are not happy with and what can be done to address these issues in order to make the environment better.

Stop, look, respond 7.4

The care environment

How would you manage the issues addressed below should a person you are caring for or offering support to find them uncomfortable? Your aim is to minimise discomfort or stress:

- The temperature of the room
- The lighting
- The noise
- Unpleasant smells
- The number of people present
- The cleanliness of the environment

If you have any concerns that their environment is causing a person discomfort or distress and you are unable to address those concerns immediately, contact a manager to seek advice on how changes can be made. If appropriate the person's family may have potentially helpful solutions that you may not have thought of.

Minimising discomfort, distress or pain

Promoting comfort both physically and psychologically is a key aspect of the role of the health or care worker. It follows therefore that you should aim to minimise discomfort, distress or pain. This can only be achieved if holistic assessment of needs has been undertaken and the plan of care is clear and person-centred. However, there may be times when you might be required to carry out aspects of care or support that the recipients may find unpleasant.

When assisting people as part of their care plan you might be required to carry out procedures or undertake activities that can also cause discomfort or pain. For example, you may be asked to help a person change their position, assist them in carrying out an activity of living or to help them to walk after they have had an operation. Your role is to minimise discomfort or pain.

Engaging the person in their care and being sensitive to the individual's needs can help to achieve this. It is essential that prior to engaging in a task or an activity you inform the person clearly (using various means).

Stop, look, respond 7.5

Providing information

A lady whose first language is not English has severe abdominal pain and the possible diagnosis is ectopic pregnancy. She needs to have surgery. Make a list of the ways in which you can be sure that this lady understands fully so she is able to provide informed consent.

Thinking cap 7.3

The use of translators

Often family members are used as translators when there is a need to explain things to people being cared for or supported.

Think about the good things and the not so good things that may be associated with using family members as translators.

In order to minimise pain or discomfort, health and social care workers are required to carry out care interventions or supporting activities with the greatest of care and sensitivity. It is essential that prior to commencing a task or touching the person in any way, you must seek their permission to do so, informing them of what you are about to do and that this may be uncomfortable or painful. Seeking consent in this way is a key component of care work and very important when you might be required to carry out activities that are unpleasant.

You could be required to enter somebody's room, and if this is the case then it is only good manners and a sign of respect that you knock prior to entering the room. Another example could be if you are asked to change a person's clothing. Then you should seek their permission, and if appropriate ask them to choose their clothing. You should explain the stages and the steps associated with the proposed procedure. By doing this the person is prepared and involved in the activity.

Always work with the person you are caring for by asking and involving them, exploring alternatives with them to determine if there may be other ways of approaching the activity, and striving to minimise or eliminate discomfort or distress.

Responding to a person's discomfort

Making appropriate and effective responses to a person's discomfort or to their pain requires effective communication. A person may tell you (verbally communicate) that they are in pain, or if they are unable to do this they could non-verbally communicate. Language is both verbal and non-verbal; our body language can confirm or contradict the words that we are actually saying.

Some people will have specific communication needs.

Stop, look, respond 7.6

Expressions

It has been suggested that there are seven types of facial expression:

1. Happiness
2. Surprise
3. Fear
4. Sadness
5. Anger
6. Disgust
7. Interest

How might a person express these through non-verbal communication?

Thinking cap 7.4

Interpreting expression

Interpreting the list of expressions described in Stop, look, respond 7.6 may be problematic in some cases as interpretation may be hindered. A person, for example, may have an injury to the face or facial nerves, or muscle weakness or a disease, such as Parkinson's disease.

You may know or suspect that someone is in pain or discomfort, for example by recognising the way they look, their body language, gestures or facial expressions; they may be sweating, pointing to an area of their body, gritting their teeth, becoming pale, crying or becoming aggressive. Then you should work with them and find a way of making them more comfortable. Acknowledge to the person that you know they are in distress and that you intend to do something about it.

Consult the person's care plan and if needed work with another worker to, for example, change their position with the person's consent. If you are unsure about what you should do then you must check with your manager or a registered healthcare professional.

Determine if there are any other factors that might be causing the person discomfort. Check environmental factors such as the person's position, noise levels, lighting, or if the person is lying in wet or soiled clothing or bed linen. Adopt agreed ways of working for addressing these issues such as the policy and procedure for moving a person, or disposing of and changing soiled bed linen or clothing.

At all times you must explain clearly and in a way that the person understands what you are doing or about to do, and why you are doing it. You should make known your actions to managers or supervisors and if appropriate document your activities.

If you have any concerns about promoting comfort and minimising pain there will be systems in your workplace that you should use to communicate your concerns, for example, during handover or at team meetings. Reporting your concerns is seen as good practice; it can improve the quality of care and support given.

Self-esteem

Being aware of and identifying the key principles of person-centred care can help to improve care provision regardless of the setting where care or support are being provided. This should effectively ensure the promotion of dignity by nurturing and supporting a person's self-respect and self-worth.

All people have a need to feel respected; this includes the need to have self-esteem. Everyone has psychological needs and these are related to feelings of self-respect, self-esteem and self-worth. People should be supported in a way that promotes confidence and self-esteem; this in turn will support and promote health and wellbeing.

Engaging in person-centred care empowers people to make choices about how their needs are met when they are unable to meet them for themselves. Respecting people as individuals and trying to help them to preserve their dignity at all times promotes person-centredness; dignity is a quality of a person's 'inner-self'. When we engage with people we should do this in a warm, sensitive and compassionate way. Engaging therapeutically and actively listening to a person's needs and concerns, responding using skills that are helpful, and providing information that is clear, accurate, meaningful and free from jargon can aid self-esteem and wellbeing. Gain the person's consent based on a sound understanding and informed choice prior to any intervention, ensuring that the person's rights in decision-making and consent are respected and upheld. This demonstrates that the care or support worker values the individual's self esteem and their wellbeing.

Personal identity

Personal identity is very closely related to dignity, self-esteem and self-worth. It is concerned with personal feelings and self-respect, providing the basis for relationships with other people. Most people have a self-image, and we wish to be treated by others in the manner we believe we deserve. Most of us have a sense of self and whether or not we are being treated in a dignified and respectful matter. It may not be possible to put this into words, but respect can be sensed. It can be very easy to damage a person's perception of their self-esteem and self-worth with a few harsh words or with physical maltreatment.

Our need to make contact with others, to feel warmth, to show affection, to love and be loved, and to show and experience pleasure or enjoyment are all closely aligned to wellbeing, including a person's sense of hope and confidence. Wellbeing, our self-esteem, our self-respect and self-worth, amongst other things, make up who we are, or our identity. All of us have different feelings, attitudes, goals and ambitions; these can also influence self-esteem and a feeling of self-worth.

Promoting wellbeing, identity and self-esteem

Promoting a person's wellbeing, their identity and self-esteem requires that the person is happy with as many aspects of their life as possible. The care or support worker must display empathy (a term that means to see things from the individual's perspective, to try to be in their shoes), be non-judgmental, listen to what the person considers important in their lives and make every effort to help them make the changes that they want.

Choice and enabling a person to make choices are closely linked to dignity and respect. The various person-centred values work in harmony; none of them can stand alone. All these values provide the person with the voice to speak up and take on as much control as possible in order to live a fulfilled life and to be as independent as possible.

Chapter summary

- Person-centred care is a comprehensive approach to assessment and services focused on an understanding of the individual's history, strengths and needs.
- In health and social care, person-centred values are those guiding principles that guide the service on how to support and assist in a person's life.
- It is important to work in a way that promotes person-centred values when supporting an individual.
- Offering person-centred care or support related to the individual's needs, wishes and preferences will help to ensure that the person is always at the centre of their care.
- One of the values associated with dignity is related to person-centred care.
- Respecting people as individuals and trying to help them to uphold their dignity at all times promotes person-centredness; dignity is a quality of a person's 'inner-self'.
- It is important to find out a person's history, preferences, wishes and needs in order to care for that person in a person-centred way.

- When a person's needs change it is important that those needs are reflected in the person's care and/or support plan.
- At the heart of a person-centred approach is the understanding that each person is unique and that they have a need to fulfil their personal potential.
- A person-centred planning process includes a dynamic discussion between the person and the service provider that identifies, considers and evaluates each person's strengths, abilities, goals and aspirations.
- Individuals might show that they are in pain or discomfort in a number of ways, and it is essential to be aware of verbal and non-verbal communication so you can recognise if they need your help and assistance to feel more comfortable.
- Personal identity is closely associated with dignity, self-esteem and self-worth.
- Person-centred values cannot work in isolation; they have to work in harmony.

Case scenario 7.1

Taff and David

Taff was in David's room supporting him to change into his gym kit so he could go with the therapist for a workout that morning. David is a 17-year-old with learning disabilities. Myfanwy, a registered nurse, walks into David's room and proceeds to ask Taff a question; Taff makes a response to Myfanwy's question, holding a conversation with her.

In this situation, the registered nurse failed to respect David's privacy and dignity; she failed to seek David's consent to enter his room; she did not even knock and wait to be invited in. Taff also failed, as he did not challenge Myfanwy. Taff is David's advocate and he should have let the nurse know that her actions were unacceptable; he should have told her to leave David's room and wait outside.
  How might you have managed this situation?

Resource file

References
Department of Health (2010) Essence of Care Communication, Promoting Health and Care Environment. London: Department of Health.
Ekman, P., Friesen, W.V., O'Sullivan, M. et al. (1987) Universals and cultural differences in the judgments of facial expressions of emotion. *Journal of Personality and Social Psychology* 53(4): 712–717.

Web resources
Care Quality Commission
Regulation 10: Dignity and respect
http://www.cqc.org.uk/content/regulation-10-dignity-and-respect

Royal College of Nursing
Dignity
https://www.rcn.org.uk/clinical-topics/nutrition-and-hydration/current-work/dignity

Chapter 8

Communication

Care certificate outcomes

1. Understand the importance of effective communication at work.
2. Understand how to meet the communication and language needs, wishes and preferences of individuals.
3. Understand how to promote effective communication.
4. Understand the principles and practices relating to confidentiality.
5. Use appropriate verbal and non-verbal communication.
6. Support the use of appropriate communication aids/technologies.

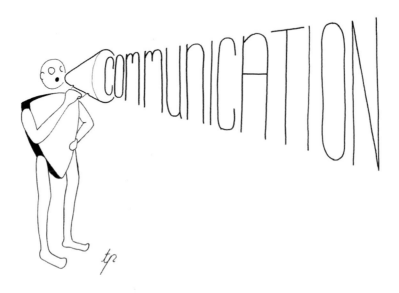

Fundamentals of Care: A Textbook for Health and Social Care Assistants, First Edition. Ian Peate.
© 2017 John Wiley & Sons Ltd. Published 2017 by John Wiley & Sons Ltd.

Take stock

Rate your current knowledge and skills prior to reading this chapter. Put a tick in the box that you think applies to you with regards to the standard being discussed:

Key:
I know this I have a good level of knowledge or skills regarding this aspect of the standard. I make use of the knowledge and skills identified on a regular basis, feeling confident in my ability and performance. I do not need a refresher.
Satisfactory My level of knowledge and standard of skills meet the criteria associated with the standard. I use the skills and knowledge from time to time. I might not always feel confident in my capability. I would benefit from a refresher.
I require a review I do not feel that I have the skills and/or the knowledge that would enable me to meet the standard in a confident and competent way. The knowledge and skills I used to have are no longer valid. I will require a refresher.
This is new to me I have never worked in a caring role before or I have never covered this topic before. I will need further training and development in this area.

Standard	Self-assessment			
Understand the importance of effective communication	☐ I know this	☐ Satisfactory	☐ I should review this	☐ This is new to me
Discuss how best to meet the communication and language needs, wishes and preferences of the people you care for or offer support to	☐ I know this	☐ Satisfactory	☐ I should review this	☐ This is new to me
Describe how to promote effective communication	☐ I know this	☐ Satisfactory	☐ I should review this	☐ This is new to me
Outline and appreciate the principles and practices relating to confidentiality	☐ I know this	☐ Satisfactory	☐ I should review this	☐ This is new to me
Describe the appropriate use of verbal and non-verbal communication	☐ I know this	☐ Satisfactory	☐ I should review this	☐ This is new to me
Highlight the need to use appropriate communication aids/technologies	☐ I know this	☐ Satisfactory	☐ I should review this	☐ This is new to me

Introduction

Being kind, being caring and being compassionate require the health and social care worker to communicate effectively – not just to communicate but to be effective in the ways in which they communicate. The way we communicate defines the way we approach the care and support we offer people.

There are many components associated with communication. This complex activity is key to successful relationships as well as to effective teamworking. One key component is listening, and this is just as important as what we say and do (verbal and non-verbal communication). The key to a positive and healthy care and support environment is communication, and when communication is effective this brings with it benefits for staff and patients.

Care, compassion and communication

There are eight components associated with care, compassion and communication. It is expected that the person being cared for can trust those providing health and social care to:

1. Work in partnership to provide collaborative care and support based on the highest standards, knowledge and competence.
2. Engage in person-centred care, empowering people to make choices about how their needs are to be met.
3. Respect people as individuals, helping them to preserve their dignity at all times.
4. Engage with the people cared for and their family or carers within their cultural environments in an acceptant and anti-discriminatory manner.
5. Provide care and support that is delivered in a warm, sensitive and compassionate way.
6. Engage with people therapeutically and actively listen to their needs and concerns, using skills that are helpful, providing information that is clear, accurate, meaningful and free from jargon.
7. Maintain confidentiality.
8. Gain informed consent prior to any intervention.

It is easy to communicate. To communicate effectively, however, is much more difficult. Much skill is required to become an effective communicator. A great deal has been written on communication, which may indicate that we often fail to communicate effectively with each other, with other health and social care professionals, and with the people to whom we offer care and support and their families.

Effective communication helps to build trust between health and social care providers and the people and their families whom they serve. Poor communication is still one of the most common reasons why people make complaints about the care and support they receive. Ineffective communication while delivering care or providing support can be made worse when health and care supporters fail to listen and respond sensitively; the outcome of this can be an overall experience that leaves a person feeling that they have not been listened to or that their individual needs have not been met. Failing to communicate effectively can damage relationships, resulting in a person's story of their experience with health and social care providers changing from one of success to one that will leave them feeling frustrated, anxious and disappointed.

Communication

At the heart of any relationship is communication, be it familial, professional, amorous or friendship. Communication can be described as a process of exchanging information, ideas, thoughts, feelings as well as emotions through a number of media, for example, speech, signals, writing or behaviour.

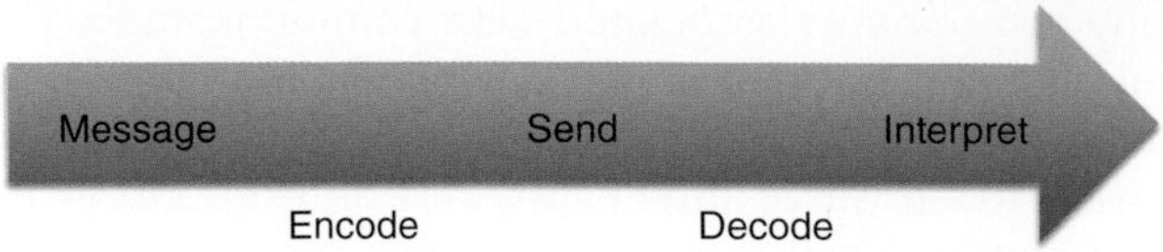

Message   Send   Interpret

Encode   Decode

Figure 8.1   The components of effective communication. *Source*: Peate, I. (2013) *The Student Nurse Toolkit*. Reproduced with permission of John Wiley & Sons, Ltd.

In order for the process of communication to be effective it requires a sender (encoder) who encodes a message and then uses a medium/channel to transmit it to the receiver (decoder), who will then decode the message. After processing information the decoder sends back feedback/reply using a medium/channel. Figure 8.1 provides a diagrammatic representation of the components of effective communication.

When communication with people is effective, health and care workers will be able to ensure that the care and support they offer is kind, compassionate and respectful, because they are listening to and acting in the person's best interests. Effective communication between health and care workers and other caregivers is critical to safe and effective care.

Thinking cap 8.1

The five Rs

Effective communication is concerned with getting the right information to the right person in the right format at the right time in the right location, all done in such a way that is easily understandable.

Think about the ways in which you communicate using the five Rs.

Types of communication

The most common means of communication is talking (verbal). However, most of how we communicate is silent (non-verbal). Gestures, tone of voice, grins, grimaces, shrugs, nods, moving away or closer, crossing arms and legs – all tell us much more than words can. Verbal communication is an important aspect of how we interact with other people but it is not the only one.

Learning to take account of these reactions is all part of developing and honing communication skills to achieve the best outcomes for people. Communication can become more difficult when we use the phone, texts or email, as we cannot see (and in some instances cannot hear) the person we are communicating with. The chosen communication channel and the style of communicating can also impact on communication effectiveness. The various types of communication and the method chosen depend on the message and the context in which it is being sent. People will use different types of communication depending on which they prefer and work best for them.

Stop, look, respond 8.1

Types of communication

Write notes and if possible give examples of where and when you have used the types of communication below.

Type of communication	Your notes
British Sign Language	
Makaton	
Braille	
Gestures	
Facial expressions	
Body position	
Assistive technology	

Verbal communication

There are several advantages that verbal communication has over other forms of communication. When we speak, for example, we are able to slow down and present points one by one. As our communication continues we are able to ensure that each point is clear and has been understood prior to moving on to the next point. This can increase the accuracy of communication.

Our use of verbal communication can be much more precise as opposed to when we use non-verbal cues. Verbal communication is enhanced when it is used with other forms of communication, for example, body language and gestures.

There are disadvantages related to the use of verbal communication, and sometimes verbal communication may not always be the best option. When verbal communication is used there is less chance of an objective record of the interaction being made; the spoken word can be quickly forgotten, particularly if there are several points to consider, so recall may be problematic. As with all types of communication there is always the possibility of miscommunication.

Non-verbal communication

This mode of communication is any kind of communication that does not involve the use of words. Non-verbal communication includes more than just facial expressions and gestures; it also includes vocal sounds that are not words, such as grunts, sighs and whimpers. Even when words are used there are non-verbal sound elements such as voice tone, pacing of speech and so on.

Stop, look, respond 8.2

The messages we send

We communicate messages to others in a number of non-verbal ways. Discreetly observe (do not breach confidentiality) the ways in which people are communicating in a non-verbal way.

Select a public place where you will be able to observe people communicating, e.g. people in a lift, a café, fast-food outlet, a football match, a railway or bus station.

Now watch and make a note on the checklist below of examples of non-verbal behaviour. Are you able to explain what the people you observed were communicating non-verbally?

	Context (when, where)	Describe the non-verbal behaviours	An explanation of what is being communicated
Person 1			
Person 2			
Person 3			

Cues

How we dress can also be a type of non-verbal communication. When a nurse wears a uniform, for example, this is communicating an important message even before a word has been said: the uniform acts as a cue. Cues carry messages, so too does their absence. In some settings failing to express a non-verbal cue communicates meaning.

Some non-verbal cues are based on learned cultural standards. However, there are some aspects of non-verbal communication that are universal, for example, anger, fear, sadness and surprise.

Setting

The setting where communication takes place also contributes to the meaning of words besides their literal definition; this too is considered non-verbal communication. For instance, the sign of a cross has much cultural meaning when used in a religious context; however, depicted on a road sign this means merely that there is a junction ahead.

Modifiers

There are some types of non-verbal communication that accompany words. These are known as modifiers, and they alter meanings. The speed of our speech and the pauses we insert between the spoken words form a non-verbal element to our speech, as they modify it. A slight pause or hesitation prior to uttering a word could suggest uncertainty, or could be interpreted as a request for the listener to confirm something. When there are no pauses, however, it implies that the speaker may be confident about what they are saying.

Personal space

Another form of non-verbal communication is the use of personal space. Leaning towards their listener as they speak, the speaker may suppose that they are communicating something that is personal or a secret. Subject to the social nuances of the situation, this could be taken as a sign of friendship or even an unwelcome invasion of space.

Haptics

Haptics is concerned with the use of touching when used as an element of communication. The meanings associated with touch are culture-dependent. In some societies a handshake is an acceptable means of greeting a person, in others this may be unacceptable and can be seen as an invasion of personal space and even disrespect.

Oculesics

Using the eyes, oculesics, is an important element of non-verbal communication. Eye movements can be divided into separate elements, such as the number and length of eye contacts, how many times the person blinks and pupil dilation. The cues and the interpretation of these cues will depend on the culture of the participants. A protracted stare could result in the formation of a bond of trust, or it may just as easily destroy it.

Non-verbal communication is how most of our communication occurs. When comparing the verbal and non-verbal aspects of communication between people, the non-verbal element is the greater part of how we convey messages.

 Thinking cap 8.2

Your day at work

Think about a day at work. Why did you need to communicate with others? Reflect on the different reasons for your communication and think about the verbal and non-verbal ways in which you communicated.

Working in teams

The need for teams and teamworking is a key element of health and social care provision. Teams, as opposed to individuals, can bring together the skills, experiences and disciplines needed to support people who use health and social care services.

Members of teams who work well together, whether in community mental health, hospitals, primary care and so on, will experience lower levels of stress. A reduction in stress levels can lead to a greater emphasis on quality service provision. A team is a group of individuals working together to deliver services; they are united by a common purpose and are committed to achieving common objectives. Working in teams allows people from different areas, with different roles and perhaps from different organisations, to work together.

Within health or social care you will be working with a multidisciplinary team. A multidisciplinary team is a group of health or social care workers and professionals who are members of different disciplines, each provides a specific service to service users. An important aspect of multidisciplinary teamwork and providing health or social care services is multi-agency working. Multi-agency working is about different services, agencies and teams of professionals working together to provide the services that meet the needs of those using the service.

Working with others can occur formally and informally. Formal communication is the type of communication that is likely to be used when in the working environment, when you and other workers interact. Informal communication is generally used with your friends and family members. When engaging in informal communication you might be using words that are familiar, dialect or slang. The method of communication that you use should always be appropriate for the person and situation.

For relationships to be successful open two-way communication is vital. Relationships that are based on trust and understanding from the outset will provide a foundation for good care and support. When communication is poor this can lead to confusion and distress. Exchanging information through communication is not always easy. If the information being shared is incorrect or confusing then this can result in mistakes being made, which can, in turn, result in poor quality care.

Thinking cap 8.3

Working with others

Think of a time when you have been at handover, a team meeting or an encounter where you were working with other health or care workers. Can you think about any cues from any individual that came from unspoken messages, such as their body language, facial expressions or gestures? Recognising the unspoken messages can help you to become more self-aware.

Communication and language needs

Finding out about a person's communication and language needs and preferences is a key aspect of your role. Effective communication occurs when the right method is used to transmit a message, so it can be received and understood. Health and social care workers need to know about a range of communication methods. You are required to identify the communication and language needs, wishes and preferences of the people with whom you work and interact.

As is the case with wider society, health and social care settings are used by people who come from a diverse range of backgrounds and who may wish or need to communicate in different ways.

You can find out about each individual's language needs, wishes and preferences by:

- Asking if they have any particular language or communication needs.
- Seeking out information about service users with regards to speech and language issues, learning difficulties, disabilities (e.g. hearing or visual impairment) or physical conditions (e.g. stroke) that could impact on a person's ability to communicate.
- Being aware that a person's culture, ethnicity and nationality can affect their language preferences and needs.
- Making observations of people who use the services provided to see how they use their communication and language skills.
- Asking others such as your supervisor/manager or specialist professionals, for example speech and language therapists, occupational therapists and social workers, for information, advice and support about how best to communicate with those having special communication needs.

Communication aids

Touch is used to communicate with people. When communicating with people who are deaf and visually impaired, touch may be used to communicate. You may need to develop the skills required to sign information onto the person's hands in an attempt to communicate and inform.

Some of the people to whom you provide care and support may have limited communication skills. When this is the case there may be a need to use technological aids. Communication devices include:

- hearing aids;
- hearing loops;
- text phones;
- text messaging on mobile phones;
- smartphone technology;
- magnifiers.

In order to be able to understand what is being said, there are some individuals who may use word or symbol boards to supplement their speech. The listener will be able to associate the picture or word with the verbal communication.

Speech synthesisers may be the preferred method of communication for some people. These replace speech either by producing a visual display of written text or by producing synthesised speech that will express the information verbally. The majority of computers have a facility whereby voice recognition software can be purchased to translate speech to written text.

It is important always to check that whatever communication aid you are using functions properly, is clean and is in good working order. Always seek advice and support if you have any concerns regarding communication aids or technology. You may be able to seek advice for the person using the device, a senior member of staff, or the person's carer or family member.

Barriers to effective communication

Sometimes you may find that in spite of all your best efforts you are unable to communicate effectively with another person in your work setting. There are many reasons why this might happen. Knowing about different barriers to effective communication will help you to avoid potential difficulties and adapt your communication approach where this is necessary. Barriers to communication are things that interfere with a person's ability to send, receive or understand a message. A barrier is anything that gets in the way of communication.

Communication can become difficult if a listener does not appear to be interested in what the person is saying, or provides them with inadequate time to say what they want to say; these are poor listening skills. Some people may have memory problems, so it can take them a little longer to process what they are trying to communicate.

Environmental factors that impact on communication include noise, poor lighting and telephones; these can make communicating with people problematic. The person can become easily distracted in environments where there is a lot going on (Table 8.1).

 ## Stop, look, respond 8.3

Barriers to effective communication

Table 8.1 provides an extensive list of factors that may impact on effective communication. Additional factors include the use of slang and dialect (yours and the person you are caring for or offering support to).

Other factors are concerned with the use of jargon and acronyms (abbreviations). Often, jargon and acronyms only make sense to those who have specialist knowledge; people who do not have this specialist knowledge may not be able to understand the message. What jargon do you use at work? Think about the acronyms you use.

Table 8.1 Factors that can have a detrimental impact on effective communication

Barrier	Impact
Developmental progress	A person's developmental stage might limit their ability to communicate. It may also be a barrier to effective communication. If these factors are not taken into account when you choose your words or the way you talk to people this can be detrimental to the caring or supporting relationship. Avoid using long sentences, complex words or unusual phrases
Environmental issues	Noise impacts negatively on listening and concentration. When there is bad lighting this can prevent a person from noting non-verbal communication and might reduce a hearing-impaired person's ability to lip read. Environments that are either too hot or too cold will cause discomfort, and those that lack privacy deter people from expressing their feelings and concerns
Sensory deprivation and disability	Visual impairment can reduce a person's ability to see faces or read signs and leaflets. If a person has a hearing impairment this may limit conversation. Conditions such as cerebral palsy, or stroke, Down syndrome and autism may limit a person's ability to communicate verbally and non-verbally
Language and cultural differences	As the UK is a multicultural country with a mix of different ethnic groups and languages there will be a potential for misinterpretation and miscommunication
Attitude	When a health or care worker is abrupt when communicating with people due to time limits, insufficient resources or low mood, the person may feel intimidated or frustrated and not want to communicate
Limited or ineffective use of technology	When technological aids that are known to be the best way for someone to communicate are not available or are being wrongly used
Body position	Sitting too close to a person might be taken as intimidation and could make a person feel uncomfortable. Sitting too far away may come across as lack of interest or concern
Distress and emotions	When an individual is depressed, angry, aggressive or upset then their emotions could impact on their ability to think and communicate in a reasonable way
Physical/biological	When a person has a physical condition that can cause communication difficulties, such as, breathlessness, being in pain or being edentulous (having no teeth)
Not having enough time	Not giving people enough time to say what they want can make them feel rushed and unwilling to express their real wishes
Poor body language	Sitting with crossed arms or legs, poor facial expressions, poor body positioning, continuous fidgeting or looking at a watch or mobile phone can make a person less inclined to communicate
Lack of privacy	If private and confidential conversations take place where people can be overheard then this may make the person reluctant to communicate
Stereotyping and prejudicing	Making generalisations about a group of people or a person that are wrong and misleading, for example 'all older people have dementia'.

Strategies to reduce barriers to communication

We all have to do what we can to reduce any barriers to communication. Knowing as much as possible about the person you are caring for or offering support to is the most effective way to make sure that you are communicating.

Some people use a communication passport; this provides a practical and person-centred method of passing on key information about people with complex communication difficulties

Table 8.2 Indicators to support best practice for communicating

- Communication is managed effectively and sensitively, including potentially difficult communication, such as conveying bad news, dealing with complaints and resolving disputes and hostile situations
- All staff are courteous, especially when faced with challenging situations
- Staff are aware of the importance of body language and effectively use non-verbal means to facilitate communication
- Communication is adapted to meet the needs of people, carers and groups. This includes thinking about the person's emotional state, hearing, vision and other physical and cognitive abilities and developmental needs, as well as their preferred language and possible need for an interpreter or translator
- Communication is open, honest and transparent
- Staff are able to establish rapport, undertake active and empathetic listening, and are non-judgmental
- When communicating with people and carers straightforward language is used
- Initiatives are in place to assess and provide feedback on the interpersonal skills of staff, for example, audit

who cannot easily speak for themselves. The information is provided in a format that is easy to read, and it may include pictures and photographs.

Issues to think about when communicating with people face-to-face:

- Places where you give face-to-face information should have low levels of background noise; a hearing aid will amplify background noise, as well as speech. Some fluorescent strip lighting can emit a humming noise, which can be distracting to hearing aid wearers.
- When talking to people, keep your face visible and do not obscure your mouth, as some people may rely on lip reading to supplement their hearing. Try not to turn your back on someone while talking to them.
- Places where you give face-to-face information should be well lit, and if possible the seating arrangements should place the person with their back to windows or other light sources. This ensures that shadows do not fall on the staff member's face, obscuring their mouth and therefore preventing the person from reading lips.
- It is important to speak clearly and not too fast. However, shouting or over-mouthing alters the lip pattern and may not be helpful.
- When initiating any conversation, you should not assume that the person to whom you are talking wishes to be called by their first name; check how they would like to be addressed.

Indicators to support best practice for communication are highlighted in Table 8.2.

Preserving confidentiality

Confidentiality is about protecting a person's right to privacy. Confidentiality is an essential aspect of your work that respects human rights. Article 8 (Right to respect for private and family life) of the European Convention of Human Rights refers to confidentiality. Health and care workers obtain private, personal information from those who use services, their relatives or from other practitioners as part of their role. You have a duty to keep any personal information about those who use services safe, and only share this information with those who have a right to know or when a person has given their permission to disclose information about them.

People have a right to expect that information given to a health or care worker will only be used for the purpose for which it was given and that this will not be disclosed without permission. One element of privacy is that individuals have the right to control access to their own personal health information. It is unacceptable to discuss matters related to the people in your care outside of your work area, discuss a person with colleagues when you are in public and where you may be overheard, or leave records unattended where they may be read by unauthorised people.

The place where you work will have a confidentiality policy concerning the sharing of confidential information. In some organisations you might be required to sign a confidentiality agreement as part of your employment contract.

A person's notes or details must be stored in a locked cupboard and not left where unauthorised people can see them. If using computers or mobile devices these need to be protected by a password and firewall.

When possible, people should provide their consent when information is being transferred. This may not always be possible and there will be circumstances when information usually deemed confidential needs to be shared. Confidentiality may need to be breached, for example, when:

- a person is likely to harm themselves;
- a person has been, or is likely to be, involved in a serious crime;
- a person is likely to harm others;
- a health or care worker's safety is at risk;
- a child or vulnerable adult has suffered, or is at risk of suffering, significant harm.

At times you may face dilemmas regarding confidentiality, such as, not knowing what to do or if you should speak to anyone about the information you have. If this occurs speak with your manager or a senior member of staff, following the agreed ways of working.

Chapter summary

- Failing to communicate effectively can have a detrimental effect on care delivered and support offered.
- To communicate effectively requires you to understand the principles underpinning communication.
- Accepting a person unconditionally without judging them, in a genuine way with empathy and positive regard, demonstrates to the person that you care.
- Confidentiality is the cornerstone of health and social care work.
- The people you care for or offer support to should be able to expect that the information they give you will be kept confidential and shared only with their consent to help with the care they are given or are to receive.
- Sometimes disclosure may be required. If you are required to disclose any information you must seek advice from a senior colleague before doing so.

Case scenario 8.1

Daniella

Daniella, a 30-year-old woman, was admitted to a hospital medical ward for observation during the night. Daniella has learning disabilities. When Daniella was admitted to the ward, she was confused and disorientated after a series of epileptic seizures. Ever since Daniella woke early this morning she has been anxious about her money and her coat. Daniella thinks that the care staff have forgotten to give her these things back, and she is becoming more and more upset about this. Daniella is sitting outside the ward office trying to get the attention of the ward manager and that of other people who are passing by.

How would you identify Daniella's communication needs in this situation? List the factors which could be affecting Daniella's ability to communicate effectively with staff.

Think of two things that you would do to respond to Daniella's communication needs in this situation.

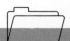

Resource file

'Hello my name is...'
http://hellomynameis.org.uk

Coalition for Collaborative Care
http://coalitionforcollaborativecare.org.uk

Chapter 9

Privacy and dignity

Care certificate outcomes

1. Understand the principles that underpin privacy and dignity in care.
2. Maintain the privacy and dignity of the individual(s) in your care.
3. Support an individual's right to make choices.
4. Support individuals in making choices about their care.
5. Understand how to support active participation.
6. Support the individual in active participation in their own care.

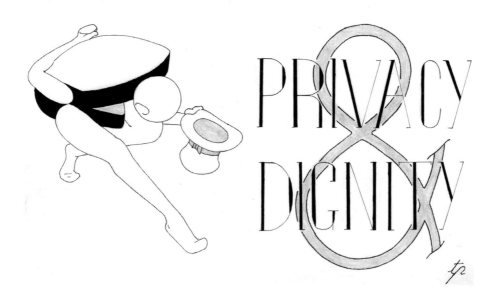

Fundamentals of Care: A Textbook for Health and Social Care Assistants, First Edition. Ian Peate.
© 2017 John Wiley & Sons Ltd. Published 2017 by John Wiley & Sons Ltd.

Take stock

Rate your current knowledge and skills prior to reading this chapter. Put a tick in the box that you think applies to you with regards to the standard being discussed:

Key:

I know this
I have a good level of knowledge or skills regarding this aspect of the standard. I make use of the knowledge and skills identified on a regular basis, feeling confident in my ability and performance. I do not need a refresher.

Satisfactory
My level of knowledge and standard of skills meet the criteria associated with the standard. I use the skills and knowledge from time to time. I might not always feel confident in my capability. I would benefit from a refresher.

I require a review
I do not feel that I have the skills and/or the knowledge that would enable me to meet the standard in a confident and competent way. The knowledge and skills I used to have are no longer valid. I will require a refresher.

This is new to me
I have never worked in a caring role before or I have never covered this topic before. I will need further training and development in this area.

Standard	Self-assessment			
Understand the principles that support privacy and dignity in care	☐ I know this	☐ Satisfactory	☐ I should review this	☐ This is new to me
Discuss how best to maintain the privacy and dignity of those in your care	☐ I know this	☐ Satisfactory	☐ I should review this	☐ This is new to me
Describe how to support a person's right to make choices	☐ I know this	☐ Satisfactory	☐ I should review this	☐ This is new to me
Outline support required to people in making choices about their care	☐ I know this	☐ Satisfactory	☐ I should review this	☐ This is new to me
Understand how people can be supported with regards to active participation in care	☐ I know this	☐ Satisfactory	☐ I should review this	☐ This is new to me
Describe the support people require to actively participate in their own care	☐ I know this	☐ Satisfactory	☐ I should review this	☐ This is new to me

Introduction

Privacy is closely related to respect. It is associated with freedom from intrusion and embarrassment, and this relates to all that is personal or sensitive with respect to an individual. Privacy underpins human dignity, is a basic human right and is the reasonable expectation of everyone (Table 9.1.).

Staff have an obligation to provide the conditions for the achievement of privacy and for dignity to flourish.

Table 9.1   Respect and dignity

Demonstrating respect to people is concerned with:

- being polite
- being thoughtful and caring
- keeping them informed
- meeting their needs
- ensuring their privacy

Respect is about treating a person as a person and not as an object of service
Dignity comes about when people are treated with respect. Often dignity is felt internally and is usually associated with a sense of:

- worth
- wellbeing
- being valued
- having a sense of purpose

Dignity is related to how people feel, how they think and behave in relation to the worth or value of themselves and others. Treating people with dignity is to treat them as being of worth, of value, in such a way that is respectful of them as valued individuals, regardless of the person's age, ethnicity, culture, gender, sexual orientation, social background, health, marital status, disability, religion or political conviction.

When positive regard is demonstrated by others towards a person as a human being and as an individual, and exhibited as courtesy, good communication, taking time and providing equal access, then this is demonstrating respect.

Recognising and supporting a person's right to privacy, dignity and respect is a key element of best practice. All people being cared for in the health and social care sectors should expect privacy, dignity and respect as their right, not as an add-on or a supplementary element of their care.

Privacy and dignity are seen as fundamental human needs, regardless of whether the person is well or ill. Being ill or requiring support and having to be cared for by others, such as a health or social care worker who may be a stranger, has the real potential to increase human dependency.

It is acknowledged, however, that there are occasions when providing privacy and dignity is difficult to achieve. This is due to the nature of caring or providing support, as this sometimes works against the achievement of total privacy and dignity. Those who provide care or offer support may have to intrude on people's most private moments and space with the intention of helping them.

Protecting information

As privacy is embedded in the rights of people then they have a right to remain alone without disturbance from others. Privacy also provides people with the right to have personal information about them held in confidence and not shared with others without their consent; this is known as privacy of information.

The law supports a person's right to privacy, for example through the Data Protection Act 1998 as well as Article 8 of the Human Rights Act 1998; it also bolsters the patient's right to privacy and dignity. When people are helped to maintain their privacy then this can promote self-control, autonomy, self-worth and dignity. To reiterate, privacy is an interlinking element of dignity.

Promoting trust and confidence and having the best interests of people at the forefront of your mind is part of providing good care and support. The health and social care worker must not discuss personal information about people where there might be the chance that it could be overheard by others; this includes using too loud a voice. Personal information includes the person's health or illness, their sexual orientation, personal history or social circumstances. People may divulge other aspects of their private life, telling you personal information; they will trust you to keep that to yourself. You should maintain confidentiality (it builds trust) unless it is necessary to pass this on for health and social care reasons.

You should only share information on a need-to-know basis, for example with other workers who are involved in the person's care. Information should not be shared with anybody else; this includes the person's family or friends, unless they give you their permission.

Disclosure

There may be occasions when a person for whom you are caring or offering support to tells you that they do not want you to share information, but you think that it is important for other workers to know in order for the person to be provided with the care and support they require. This kind of situation needs to be handled with sensitivity. It is important that you take time to explain to the person what your concerns are and the reason(s).

You should aim to try to seek an understanding over the amount and type of information that the person is willing for you to pass on. If you still feel that this is not in their best interest then speak with your manager about the issue. Your manager can help you decide whether you should tell the person that you must pass on something that is in their best interest with regard to their care and support.

There may be occasions when you may be required to disclose information given to you and this should never be taken lightly. Disclosure is only lawful and ethical if the person has given their consent for that information to be passed on, and such consent is freely and fully given. Consent to disclosure of confidential information may be:

- explicit;
- implied;
- requested by law;
- disclosed by reason of the public interest.

Disclosure with consent

Explicit consent is acquired when the person you are caring for agrees to disclosure once they have been informed of the reason for disclosure and who the information may or will be shared with. Explicit consent can be written or spoken.

Implied consent occurs when it is assumed that the person being cared for understands that their information may be shared within the healthcare team. The people to whom you offer care or provide support should be made aware of this routine of sharing of information; if there are any objections seek assistance from your manager and ensure that you record these objections clearly.

Disclosure without consent

The term 'public interest' describes the exceptional circumstances that validate overruling the rights of a person to confidentiality. The aim here is to serve a broader social concern.

Staff are allowed under common law to disclose personal information in order to prevent and support detection, investigation and punishment of a serious crime and/or to prevent abuse or serious harm to others. Each case in this instance will be judged on its merits. The following examples could include disclosing information in relation to crimes against the person:

- rape;
- child abuse;
- murder;
- kidnapping;
- injuries that are sustained from knife or gunshot wounds.

Decisions made with regards to disclosure are complex and they must take into account the public interest in ensuring confidentiality as well as the public interest in disclosure. Advice from a senior manager should be sought prior to disclosing any information.

Disclosure to third parties

If information is shared with other people and/or organisations that are not directly involved in a person's care then this is considered disclosure to a third party. If this type of disclosure is indicated then the people being cared for or offered support to must be made aware that their information could be disclosed to third parties who are involved in their care. The person may object to the use and disclosure of their information, and if this is the case then it should be clearly documented.

The government and other organisations have produced guidance regarding confidentiality; there is also advice available concerning public interest disclosure. This kind of guidance is underpinned by the legislation such as the Data Protection Act and the Human Rights Act.

Stop, look, respond 9.1

Disclosure

Every employer should have in place a procedure for raising concerns (whistleblowing procedure) to facilitate the disclosure of sensitive information. Can you locate the procedure in your place of work?

Make notes about the procedure and identify the various stages of the process.

_____
_____
_____
_____
_____

Implementing respect, privacy and dignity

When dignity is absent from care, people will feel devalued; they will lack the ability to take control and be comfortable. They can also lack confidence, be unable to make decisions for themselves, feel humiliated, embarrassed and ashamed. Dignity is the essence of care and

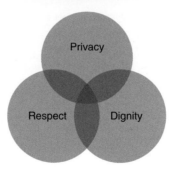

Figure 9.1   The closely intertwined interrelated connections between respect, privacy and dignity.

support, and because of this it must be at the heart of everything that is done for people. Care given and support offered should be done in such a way that it is compassionate and empathetic and given in a respectful and non-judgmental way. Each person has the right to receive high-quality care that is safe, effective and respects their privacy and dignity; all of these issues are closely interrelated and intertwined (Figure 9.1).

Stop, look, respond 9.2

Respect, dignity and privacy

Write notes on the following:
   Respect is....

_____
_____
_____
_____

   Dignity is.....

_____
_____
_____

   Privacy is.....

_____
_____
_____

A commitment to the delivery of care with privacy and dignity can be demonstrated in many ways; for example, the provision of gender-appropriate accommodation for people and safeguarding them when they are at their most vulnerable. Table 9.2 outlines some of the ways in which promoting a person's dignity can be achieved.

Table 9.2 Some of the ways the health and care worker can promote a person's dignity

- Providing people with their own clothes
- Assisting people to dress in their own clothes appropriate to the time of day and with respect to their individual preferences
- Ensuring that if the person is wearing hospital clothes, for example, a hospital gown, this protects their modesty
- Grooming residents as they wish to be groomed
- Combing a person's hair and styling it as they wish, shaving the person or trimming their beard according to their preference, cleaning and clipping nails
- Assisting people to attend to activities of their own choosing
- Promoting a person's independence and dignity when dining, for example, avoiding the use of plastic cutlery and paper/plastic dishware, providing napkins instead of bibs, ensuring the dining room is conducive to pleasant dining
- Respecting a person's private space and their property
- Not changing a radio or television channel without the person's permission
- Knocking on doors and requesting permission to enter; closing doors as requested by the person; always making your presence known
- Not moving or inspecting a person's personal possessions without permission
- Respecting a person's social status by speaking with them respectfully, and listening carefully to what the person is saying
- Treating a person with respect, for example, addressing that person with a name of their choice, and not excluding people from conversations
- Not discussing the person in a community setting
- Focusing on people as individuals when talking with them and addressing them as individuals when providing care and support

Stop, look, respond 9.3

Maintaining dignity

Review the list in Table 9.2. This should not be seen as a comprehensive list, and there are many other ways in which dignity can be maintained. Provide details of ways in which you maintain dignity at work when offering care to people or providing support to them.

_____
_____
_____

Employees must adhere to agreed ways of working, behaving in such a way that this promotes openness and shows unconditional positive regard. You should give due consideration to the manner in which people are treated and you should not discriminate against people. The manner in which staff relate to the people for whom they are caring or offering support has the potential to positively or negatively impact on the person's sense of self and wellbeing.

Thinking cap 9.1

Wellbeing

Think about those things that make you feel good – it may be the clothes you are wearing, the way people give you compliments, the food you are eating, the company you are in. There are many things that can boost our sense of wellbeing. Think also about the things you say or do when you work with people and how this can impact on a person's self-esteem.

Implementing care that is based on dignity and respect means that the person providing care or offering support must know what the person's needs are. You must know the person's likes and dislikes from a holistic perspective – their strengths and weaknesses, wants and needs. You must ensure, however, that the person (unless unable to) should make their own decisions about their life.

Aiming to ensure that people feel safe and are comfortable requires effort. You have to engage with them – talk with them, find out more about them, look at their care plan to determine how in different situations they want to be treated. Explore and encompass with the person their individual values, beliefs and personal relationships.

Some people want their carer, family members or friends to be involved in their care or kept up to date about their care and support. Conversely, others will want to retain entirely for themselves the responsibility for disclosing information or about how far they want to have others involved in their personal care or life. You will only be able to determine this if you ask the person what they want, get to know them and act on their behalf. Whatever choice the person makes should be respected and you should support them in that choice. This could mean, however, that there will be times when you have to act sensitively in challenging the assumptions that others have made, your first interest is the person you are caring for.

113

Stop, look, respond 9.4

Paternalism

What do you understand by paternalism? See if you can find a definition of this term.

Paternalism occurs when the health or social care worker does not respect the person's right to autonomy. They act as if they know what is best as opposed to what the person being cared for or being offered support to wishes or wants. Give an example of how you (or another) have acted in a paternalistic manner.

Paternalism is based upon the health or social care worker's beliefs about what is in the best interest of the person. This principle (paternalism) is very closely associated with the application of power over people.

Paternalism disempowers the person.

Personal space

Another element of ensuring that privacy, dignity and respect are valued is to ensure that a person's personal space is respected and protected.

An awareness of proximity, or the amount of personal space that a person requires, is also an important feature of effective communication (Chapter 8 discusses this further):

- Being physically close to someone can be reassuring and may be seen as accepting the person.
- However, it might make the person feel uncomfortable and vulnerable.
- People require less personal space when they have a close, trusting relationship.

We all have our own idea, our view, of what constitutes our personal space so it is important to find out from the people we care for what is comfortable for them. Wherever you work, there will be issues about personal space, privacy and dignity. In order to ensure you understand the issues, you should talk about them with other people you work with or your manager.

The care environment can be defined as an area where care takes place; this could be a building (a person's home, hospital) or a vehicle (e.g. an ambulance). The personal environment may be regarded as the immediate area in which a person receives care. For example, this can be in a person's home, a consulting room, hospital bed space, prison, or any treatment/clinic area.

You will be required to respect and protect the individual's personal space (environment) according to their wishes. Policies or plans should be in place to avoid disturbing or interrupting people, for example requesting and awaiting an invitation to enter a person's personal space; entering their personal area only when given permission to do so – this includes their room or entry to their home. Protecting a person's space also means that people are afforded privacy, for example using curtains, screens, providing blankets and appropriate clothing, and ensuring that they are not cared for in a mixed sex environment (i.e. a mixed sex ward).

Informed choice and choosing options

The choices that people make are shaped by their background, values, culture, religion or life experiences. Everyone has the right to weigh up and take risks that they consider will make their life enjoyable and worthwhile.

When working with other people, those to whom you offer care or support have the right to make their own choices and to take any risks once they understand all the information available and are fully aware of the risks. Enabling people to take risks means that you will have to support the individual to identify and assess their own risks and then allow them to take the risks that they choose. As a person providing care or offering support, you can give your view but it is the individual's right to choose.

When applying a person-centred approach this requires you to involve the individual in the planning of their care and support them as much as possible. There may be times, however, when someone is unhappy with decisions that have been made on their behalf or with the choices that they are offered. People have a right to complain, and if you have to you may be required to support the person to access and follow the complaints procedure.

Making choices and selecting options is a key aspect of the NHS Constitution, a document produced in England that sets out the principles and values of the NHS. It sets out rights to which those who use services, public and staff, are entitled to, pledges that the NHS is committed to achieve, together with responsibilities in order to ensure that the NHS operates equitably and effectively. Engaging in person-centred care, speaking with people, and getting to know them can empower them to make choices about how their needs are met when they are unable to meet them for themselves.

Offering people choice is very closely aligned to the promotion of dignity. All individuals should be fully involved in any decision that affects their care. This will include any personal decisions they make such as what they want to eat or do not want to eat, what they wish to wear and what time they choose to go to bed as well as wider decisions concerning their care or support.

People will only be able to make choices if they have the information available to them. The information, however, has to be made available in a manner that the person can understand. They will also need to know about the options they have available, the potential risks and the possible consequences of the choice that they make. When all of this is made available it is termed an informed choice. Even if a person has all of the information available, decisions concerning choice and options can be challenging.

There are many ways in which you can help the person to make an informed choice but this too can be difficult. Acting as the person's advocate you can offer an explanation or information, introduce the person to others who can share their experiences, or seek the help and assistance

Thinking cap 9.2

Information and making decisions

Think about how you decide how much information, the level of information, the type of information, and the format in which you provide it to people in order for them to make an informed decision.

of specialist workers, friends or relatives. You can only do this, however, with the permission of the person you are caring for or offering support to.

There may be some people who are unable to understand and retain (recall, recollect) the information they have been given in order to make a decision or to communicate their choice. They may lack the mental capacity to make the decision. On a day-to-day basis the person may be able to make choices about what they want to do that day, what they want to wear and what they want to eat; however, they may not be able to make complex decisions regarding their finances or their health (medical issues). When you are faced with circumstances that you are not completely sure about and they concern the person's capacity, it is important that you obtain further advice or guidance.

Assessing risk

Every decision we make, every choice we make brings with it potential risk. In keeping people safe and preventing danger, harm and accidents the law requires those who provide services to undertake risk assessments. People receiving care or support should have a risk assessment undertaken as part of their care, support, rehabilitation or treatment plan.

There are a number of risk assessments available and they provide guidance on how people can be kept safe. A risk assessment contains information on potential hazards associated with the care and support provided and any actions that may need to be taken to control any risks. Information contained in a risk assessment will take account of the person's daily care and support, for example, their personal hygiene or mobility and how best to protect them and others from possible harm.

When caring for people or offering them support, any new activity that is to be introduced should be assessed using the five steps of risk assessment. Figure 9.2 considers the cyclical approach to risk assessment using the five steps.

Stop, look, respond 9.5

Risks

Take some time to think about the risks that are evident in your organisation and make a list of them; it might be a good idea to sit with your manager to complete this task. Think about severity of risk and how these risks might be minimised or alleviated.

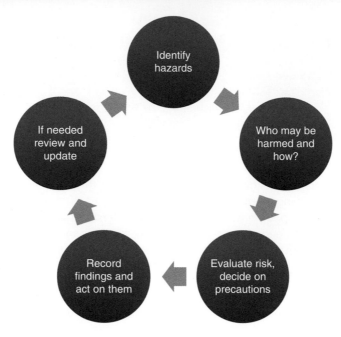

Figure 9.2   Risk assessment: a cyclical approach.

Equality and diversity

Each of us has a duty not to discriminate against those we care for or offer support to, and the staff we work with. Agreed ways of working also demand that we adhere to equal opportunities and equality and human rights legislation. Health and social care organisations have a responsibility, under the Public Sector Equality Duty, to eliminate discrimination and advance equality.

The terms equality and diversity are sometimes used interchangeably although they are not the same. Equality is concerned with creating a fairer society, where everyone can participate and has the opportunity to fulfil their potential. Diversity literally means difference, and is about recognising the individual and groups as having differences, treating people as individuals and placing positive value on diversity.

Eliminating prejudice and discrimination and promoting independence can ensure that services delivered are personal, respectful and fair. This requires us all to tackle discrimination in the workplace. An equalities approach to service provision understands who we are, based on social categories such as gender, race, disability, age, social class, sexuality and religion, and impacts on our life experiences.

Stereotyping is to have an opinion about a group and then applying this to anyone who belongs to this group. Prejudice means to prejudge; it could mean that you do not like someone just because of the group that they belong to. In a modern health and social care system there is no place for prejudice or stereotyping of any type and they should always be challenged.

Stop, look, respond 9.6

Stereotyping and prejudice

Make a list of some of the stereotypes that may be associated with people in different groups. Two have already been listed; add some more to this list.

Group	Stereotypes
Elderly people	They are all incontinent
Deaf people	They are educationally challenged

In order to make sure that you do not allow prejudice and stereotyping to have a negative impact on the quality of your work, reflecting on your own attitudes and beliefs is key. Reflection is a systematic activity that can help you, using a process, to think about your experiences in a way that is critical. It can help you to explore what you could do differently, develop or change the next time a similar situation arises.

Stop, look, respond 9.7

Reflection

Think about an incident or an issue that has arisen recently. Using the proposed reflective approach below make comments on the five points listed (remember to maintain confidentiality):

1. What happened?
2. What went well?
3. What didn't go so well?
4. What could you do to improve?
5. How will you put this into practice next time?

A key attribute when working in a health or social care setting is that you need to be positive, unbiased and demonstrate that you have respect for attitudes and beliefs that other people hold. This is particularly essential when they are not the same as your own. Your role is to give consideration to the physical, emotional and spiritual wellbeing of people and permit them, as far as possible, to live their life the way that they choose in health and in illness.

Dependence ←-- → Independence

Figure 9.3   Dependence/independence continuum.

Promoting independence

A person's independence is considered on a continuum that ranges from complete dependence to complete independence (Figure 9.3). Using this continuum can help the care or support worker decide what interventions (if any) will be needed to lead to increased independence as well as what ongoing support may be needed to offset any dependency that exists. The person's dependence and independence should be reviewed throughout the care plan.

Encouraging independence and promoting active participation is a way of working that supports an individual's right to make decisions. The person can decide to take part in activities (or decline to do so) and this can then encourage relationships that can lead to independence. The person is an active partner in their own care or support, as opposed to being a grateful passive recipient. It is the person who is the expert, not the person assisting; it is the person who knows best the way of life that matters to them, whereas the care or support worker listens and at all times takes this into account.

Thinking cap 9.3

Involving people in their care

Think of occasions where you could involve the person more in their care or the support you offer them as opposed to making assumptions about their needs.

When a person takes control of their care (or is assisted to) or what they want to be supported with, this will help that person to construct their own identity and boost their self-esteem. Issues associated with equality and diversity should also be considered when promoting independence, providing the person with an equal opportunity to achieve their goals and aspirations, valuing their diversity and helping them to identify solutions that will work for them.

Chapter summary

- Privacy provides people with the right to have personal information about them held in confidence and not shared with others without their consent.
- There may be occasions when confidentiality can be breached, but you must seek advice about this prior to divulging.
- People should be helped (if needed) to understand the care and treatment choices that are available to them.
- They should be given the opportunity to express their views and be involved in making decisions about their care.
- They have a right to privacy, dignity and independence and this should be respected.
- Those providing care or offering support should take the person's views and experiences into account in the way the service is devised, developed, delivered and evaluated.

- People have the right to weigh up and take risks that they consider will make their life enjoyable and worthwhile.
- In a contemporary health and social care system there is no place for prejudice or stereotyping, and these should always be challenged.
- We all have a duty not to discriminate against those we care for or offer support to and the staff we work with.
- Promoting independence and encouraging active participation is a way of working that supports an individual's right to make decisions.

119

Case scenario 9.1

Renuka

Renuka is a co-worker and she was diagnosed with depression about a year ago. She did not tell anyone about this until three months ago, when she revealed what she was experiencing and the treatment that she was getting from her doctor and therapist. A month ago she was signed off on sick leave. Renuka returned to work last week; however, she tells you she is overwhelmed. She is determined, though, to carry on with her work.

What support can you offer Renuka?

Resource file

NHS England Confidentiality Policy
http://www.england.nhs.uk/wp-content/uploads/2013/06/conf-policy-1.pdf

NHS Constitution
https://www.gov.uk/government/uploads/system/uploads/attachment_data/file/480482/NHS_Constitution_WEB.pdf

Chapter 10

Fluids and nutrition

Care certificate outcomes

1. Understand the principles of hydration, nutrition and food safety.
2. Support individuals to have access to fluids in accordance with their plan of care.
3. Support individuals to have access to food and nutrition in accordance with their plan of care.

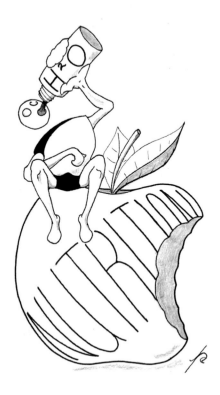

Fundamentals of Care: A Textbook for Health and Social Care Assistants, First Edition. Ian Peate.
© 2017 John Wiley & Sons Ltd. Published 2017 by John Wiley & Sons Ltd.

Take stock

Rate your current knowledge and skills prior to reading this chapter. Put a tick in the box that you think applies to you with regards to the standard being discussed:

Key:

I know this
I have a good level of knowledge or skills regarding this aspect of the standard. I make use of the knowledge and skills identified on a regular basis, feeling confident in my ability and performance. I do not need a refresher.

Satisfactory
My level of knowledge and standard of skills meet the criteria associated with the standard. I use the skills and knowledge from time to time. I might not always feel confident in my capability. I would benefit from a refresher.

I require a review
I do not feel that I have the skills and/or the knowledge that would enable me to meet the standard in a confident and competent way. The knowledge and skills I used to have are no longer valid. I will require a refresher.

This is new to me
I have never worked in a caring role before or I have never covered this topic before. I will need further training and development in this area.

Standard	Self-assessment			
Understand the principles of hydration, nutrition and food safety	☐ I know this	☐ Satisfactory	☐ I should review this	☐ This is new to me
Explain the importance of good nutrition and hydration in maintaining a person's health and wellbeing	☐ I know this	☐ Satisfactory	☐ I should review this	☐ This is new to me
Describe the signs and symptoms of poor nutrition and hydration	☐ I know this	☐ Satisfactory	☐ I should review this	☐ This is new to me
Explain how to promote adequate nutrition and hydration	☐ I know this	☐ Satisfactory	☐ I should review this	☐ This is new to me
Describe how people can be supported with regards to hydration and nutrition	☐ I know this	☐ Satisfactory	☐ I should review this	☐ This is new to me
Describe how to ensure that drinks and nutritional products can be made available to those who have restrictions on their movement/ mobility	☐ I know this	☐ Satisfactory	☐ I should review this	☐ This is new to me

Introduction

Food and fluids are necessary for life; they are also a source of great pleasure, with important social, cultural and religious functions. Mealtimes are not just about the food we eat, they are also about who you eat with, where you eat your meal and if it is a comfortable place to be.

What we eat is vital to our health and wellbeing and to how we look, feel and function. It is important that people have a diet that is safe to eat and contains all the nutrients that they need.

Thinking cap 10.1

Places to eat

Take some time and think about the places where you like to go to eat.

Why do you like to go there?
Who do you like to go there with?
What kind of food do you like to eat there?

A great deal of research has been undertaken and published on the importance of a healthy balanced diet and lifestyle to the health and wellbeing of people and communities. A healthy diet can help to reduce the risk of heart disease, stroke, diabetes, obesity and a number of other medical conditions. It can also have a positive impact on a person's social and psychological functioning, and on how they look and feel.

Promoting good nutritional care is everyone's business. Good nutrition and adequate hydration are of vital importance for people recovering from illness, or for those who may be at risk of malnutrition. Food safety is essential when preparing and handling food.

Food and drink safety

Safe practice is a key element of the role of the health or social care worker, and this extends to the safe preparation and handling of food. There are a number of legislative measures and regulations in place to support health and safety at work with regards to food safety. These aim to protect those at work, those people using services and the wider public.

The Food Safety Act in England (the Food Hygiene Regulations in Scotland) covers the preparation, storage and service of food and requires the registration of food businesses whether they are run for profit or not. A 'food business' includes care homes, hospitals, prisons, canteens and clubs. Regulators, for example the Care Quality Commission (CQC), require that care services ensure that the food and drink they provide is handled, stored, prepared and delivered in a way that aligns to the requirements of the Act. In England the local authority has a responsibility to enforce the law through Environmental Health and Trading Standards. The Food Standards Agency (FSA) has the power to intervene if local authorities have failed to meet the requirements and also in emergency situations.

Food safety legislation requires any organisation that handles food to ensure that all of its activities are carried out in a hygienic manner; organisations must comply with the law. A criminal offence is committed if an organisation supplies food that is unsafe or harmful to human health. There are clear minimum requirements for food hygiene and safety.

Food safety measures are associated with the steps that have to be taken to prevent food from becoming contaminated. The overriding aim for applying food safety processes is to prevent people you care for or offer support to from becoming ill from food that has been contaminated.

In an organisation such as a care home, large numbers of people could become ill if food safety measures are not followed in the appropriate manner. It is essential that at all times high standards of food hygiene are maintained. Illnesses as a result of poor practice can range from mild to severe.

It is possible for people to become ill from eating food that tastes normal and looks safe, as not all substances and objects that may cause harm or illness can be seen. Because of this it is easy to spread bacteria. The health and social care worker must ensure that the food they provide for people is safe to eat, irrespective of whether they are simply making a snack or are regularly involved in preparing meals.

Food must be prepared and stored in ways that prevent it becoming contaminated with things that have the potential to result in harm or cause illness. The best way to avoid food risks, such as food poisoning, is to make sure that high standards of food hygiene are maintained when storing, handling and preparing food. Knowledge of food hygiene is vital for any person who handles food so that they are able to avoid harm. You will need to know about the steps required to prevent risks associated with food poisoning.

Allergenic hazards

Substances in food that can cause an allergy – allergenic substances – can result in extreme reactions if a person is allergic to that particular ingredient or substance, such as nuts, eggs, shellfish, milk or wheat.

Anaphylaxis is a serious and potentially life-threatening allergic reaction to an allergy. Symptoms may include hives, runny nose, sneezing, swollen hands, feet or eyelids, itchy mouth, throat or eyes, stomach cramps with vomiting or diarrhoea, difficulty with breathing, and/or collapse and unconsciousness.

Foods that contain allergens should always be kept and prepared separately from foods that do not.

Physical hazards

Food may become unsafe to eat through physical contamination, as when something falls into or onto food. Physical hazards include objects that may be harmful, for example bones or fragments of packaging. They may not cause food poisoning but they might cause choking. These items may be present in food that has been bought or introduced whilst preparing food.

Where possible you should check for these physical hazards and remove them.

Microbiological/bacterial hazards

These include dangerous microorganisms (pathogens) that can cause disease, for example food-borne illnesses (caught by eating contaminated food). Eating food that has been contaminated with harmful microorganisms may result in food-borne illnesses.

Harmful microorganisms can be found in raw foods, which need to be cooked in order to remove the pathogens, or in the human gut (bowel), nose and mouth, pathogens from which can be transferred to food during storage, handling and preparation.

Three types of microorganisms can contaminate food causing food-borne illness:

- bacteria;
- viruses;
- parasites.

Fungi are another group of microorganisms that are present in the form of yeast and moulds. These yeasts and moulds will spoil food and generally they will not cause food-borne illnesses, although some produce toxins that can cause serious illness, especially in people who are immunocompromised.

To avoid microbiological risks, effective food safety principles should be followed, protecting food from being contaminated with bacteria. These bacteria can come from sources such as:

- raw food;
- humans;
- pests;
- waste products;
- contaminated water;
- the environment.

Chemical hazards

These include insecticides, pesticides, weedkillers (these may be used by farmers) or cleaning chemicals that if ingested (eaten) could be harmful, for example pesticides that are attached to fresh fruit and vegetables, or cleaning products sprayed onto prepared foods. If cleaning chemicals are not stored correctly they have the potential to contaminate food; these products must be controlled appropriately. Transfer of cleaning chemicals to food may occur in a variety of ways; these include: chemical residues transferred to food containers; failure to wash chemicals from surfaces after cleaning; leakage of chemicals into a food storage area if the chemicals are not stored correctly.

All fruit and vegetables must be washed prior to preparation and the spraying of cleaning products around food should be avoided. Read and follow instructions and ensure procedures are followed when using cleaning products. Store chemicals securely and separately from food or food packaging.

 Stop, look, respond 10.1

Food safety hazards

In your place of work have a look around the food preparation areas and identify as many hazards (actual or potential) as you can. Group them into the boxes below:

Physical	Bacterial/microbiological	Chemical

Think about ways in which you might prevent them.

Protecting people

Some people, due to a variety of reasons, are more prone (or vulnerable) to certain bacteria that can cause them illness, and because of this the symptoms these people experience may be more severe. Groups of people who are deemed more vulnerable due an impaired immune system can include:

- babies, toddlers, children and teenagers;
- pregnant and breastfeeding women;
- elderly people;
- those living on a low income;
- people in prison;
- people in hospital.

Protecting people is your first concern, and applying food safety measures can help with this. When handling food you will be required to:

- always wash your hands;
- wear clean clothes;
- wear an apron (personal protective equipment) if handling unwrapped food;
- remove your watch or jewellery if you are wearing them;
- tie back your hair and wear a hat or hairnet if appropriate (seek advice if unsure).

You must not do the following:

- smoke;
- eat or drink;
- touch your face, cough or sneeze over food.

You must cover any cuts with a highly coloured waterproof dressing.

Figure 10.1 outlines some of the principles associated with food hygiene.

You must wash your hands (Figure 10.2) prior to touching any food, particularly ready-to-eat food, and after doing any of the following:

- using the toilet;
- coming back from your break;
- touching raw meat, poultry, fish, eggs or unwashed vegetables;
- touching a cut or changing a dressing;
- touching or emptying bins;
- carrying out any cleaning;
- touching a phone, light switches or door handles.

Personal protective equipment in food hygiene

Ensuring that bacteria and other contaminants are not introduced into food requires you to implement a number of strategies. The use of personal protective equipment (PPE) to maintain hygiene when handling food and drink will be required. The type of PPE needed will be related to the task being undertaken. Types of PPE include:

- disposable aprons;
- hats or hairnets;
- disposable gloves.

Hairnets are worn to prevent loose hairs from falling into food. Hair constantly falls out and as well as with dandruff this can result in the contamination of food. Long hair should be tied back and a suitable hair covering, such as a hairnet, worn when food is being prepared.

Disposable aprons are used to protect food from any bacteria that could be present on the clothing of the health or care worker. Aprons should be worn when carrying out activities involving food, such as when assisting or offering support to people to eat or when serving food.

Working with food?
What you need to know
before you start

It is easy for you to spread bacteria to food without realising.
These bacteria are invisible and could make customers ill.
Your personal hygiene is important.

This is what you need to do to keep food safe:

Before you start working with food

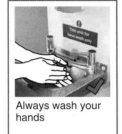

Always wash your hands

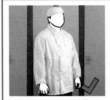

Wear clean clothes

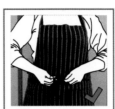

Wear an apron if handling unwrapped food

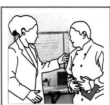

Tell your manager if you have vomiting or diarrhoea and do not work with food

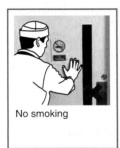

Take off your watch and jewellery

It is a good idea to tie hair back and wear a hat or hairnet

When you are working with food

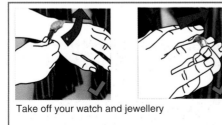

No smoking

No eating or drinking

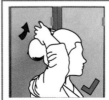

Avoid touching your face, coughing or sneezing over food

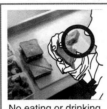

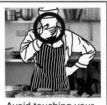

Cover cuts with a brightly coloured waterproof dressing

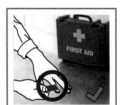

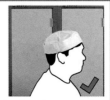

Figure 10.1 Food hygiene. Source: https://www.food.gov.uk/sites/default/files/multimedia/pdfs/publication/sfbb-workingwithfd-0513.pdf. Reproduced under OGL.

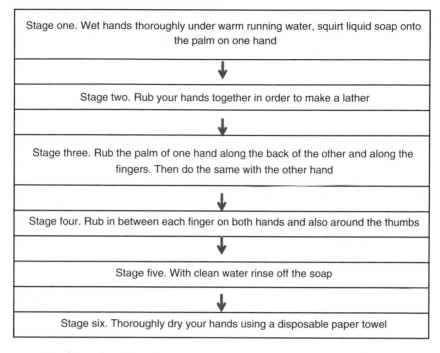

Figure 10.2   Food hygiene, hand washing.

Gloves provide a physical barrier between the health and social care worker's hands and all other surfaces. It is not a requirement to wear gloves; however, it is a requirement that those who handle food maintain a high standard of personal hygiene, meaning that hands must be washed thoroughly. When gloves are worn, then they must be changed on a frequent basis. This is important as the warm, moist conditions inside the gloves can promote the growth of bacteria.

Stop, look, respond 10.2

Disposal of food waste

It is important to ensure that food waste is disposed of safely and in a timely manner. Waste and food that is unfit for consumption must not be allowed to build up in those areas where food and drink are prepared as this can attract pests and rodents if it is not disposed of correctly.
   In the place where you work determine the policy for the disposal of all waste food.
   What types of bins are in use? How often are they emptied?

Nutrition and hydration

Promoting good nutrition and hydration in the maintenance of health and wellbeing is an important activity undertaken by the health and social care worker. Food and drink have to provide the nutrients that the body requires to function effectively and prevent illness or disease. To remain healthy a balanced diet is required.

Table 10.1   Components of a balanced diet

Component	Discussion	Example
Carbohydrates	Carbohydrates provide most of the energy the body requires. Some of this energy is needed for the basic actions that keep us alive, known as the basal metabolic rate, such as, maintaining the heartbeat, facilitating breathing, keeping the blood circulating, and the production of hormones and enzymes and for new tissues	Bread, beans, potatoes, rice or pasta
Vitamins	Vitamins provide the body with support for a number of functions, including helping the blood to clot, maintaining an efficient immune system and facilitating the absorption of energy from foods	Good sources of vitamins can be found in fruit, soybeans and vegetables

Minerals	Minerals help the body to grow, develop and stay healthy. They are required to perform a range of functions, from building strong bones to the transmission of nerve impulses. Some minerals are used to make hormones or to maintain a normal heartbeat
	    Calcium helps to build strong bones and teeth. Iron (a mineral) is needed to transport oxygen from the lungs to the rest of the body
	    Potassium maintains muscle activity and helps keep the nervous system working properly
	    Zinc assists with maintaining an effective immune system. The immune system helps to fight off illnesses and infections. It also helps with cell growth and helps wounds to heal
		Milk products are good providers of calcium; other minerals can be found in vegetables such as broccoli. Liver, shellfish, lentils and beans contain high levels of iron

Fibre	Fibre promotes healthy bowel activity, helping to remove waste products from the body Fibre can be insoluble (this helps keep a healthy bowel and avoid constipation promoting the movement of food through the gut) or soluble (which helps to promote healthy gut bacteria and lower cholesterol by slowing down digestion)	Fruit, vegetables, wholemeal bread, nuts and seeds are high in fibre
Protein	Proteins are the building blocks of the body. Protein is important for the body's cells and tissues to be repaired and replaced. Protein is a major part of the skin, muscles, organs and glands	Found in milk products as well as in poultry, fish, eggs, dairy products, nuts, seeds, and legumes like black beans and lentils

Good nutrition has a significant impact on a person's general wellbeing. Poor nutrition can have an effect on a person's energy levels, how alert they are, their ability to mobilise and mobilise safely, healing and recovery. Understanding more about nutrition, malnutrition and hydration along with knowing what types of food and drink are preferred by the people you care for, will enable you to encourage them to eat and drink the right things that will help them stay well or recover if they are ill. The components of a balanced diet are outlined in Table 10.1.

The Eatwell plate

The Eatwell plate defines the UK government's advice on a healthy balanced diet. It is a visual representation of how different foods will contribute towards a healthy balanced diet. The size of the segments for each food group is in alignment with government's recommendations for a diet that will provide all of the nutrients required for a healthy adult or child over the age of 5.

The Eatwell plate (Figure 10.3) is based on the five food groups; this makes healthy eating easier to understand and provides a visual representation of the types and proportions of foods that are needed for a healthy balanced diet.

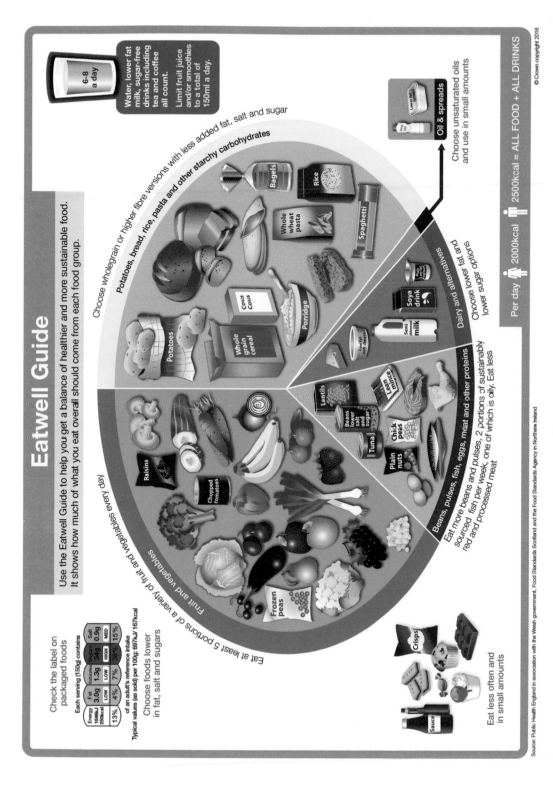

Figure 10.3 The Eatwell plate. *Source:* Public Health England in association with the Welsh Government, Food Standards Scotland and the Food Standards Agency in Northern Ireland.

Selecting foods from within the main food groups will add to the range of nutrients consumed. These will include:

- plenty of fruit and vegetables;
- plenty of bread, rice, potatoes, pasta and other starchy foods;
- some milk and dairy foods;
- some meat, fish, eggs, beans and other non-dairy sources of protein.

Foods and drinks high in fat and/or sugar are not essential to a healthy diet and as such should be consumed only in small amounts.

Hydration

It is important to stay hydrated; the body depends on water to survive. Every cell, tissue and organ in the body needs water to function effectively. The body requires water to maintain its temperature, remove waste and to lubricate joints. Water is needed for good health.

When a person does not have enough fluid the body will be unable to carry out basic processes that allow it to function correctly. As a person ages their thirst sensation can lessen, and as a result of this they may not drink enough. Those who may be unable fully to mobilise or those who become less mobile can find it difficult to get up to get themselves a drink.

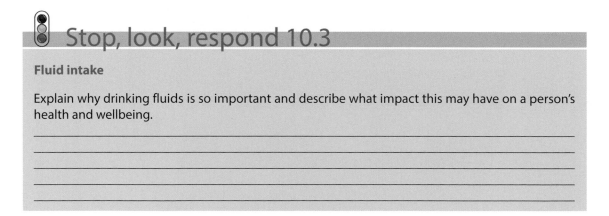

Stop, look, respond 10.3

Fluid intake

Explain why drinking fluids is so important and describe what impact this may have on a person's health and wellbeing.

_____
_____
_____
_____
_____

The average amount of water that a person needs to drink is 30 millilitres per kilogram of body weight per day. However, in warm weather or if person has an infection, this will increase. With insufficient fluids the person may have problems with:

- digesting food and enabling nutrients to be absorbed;
- enabling blood to circulate around the body;
- removing waste products via urine and faeces;
- keeping cells and tissues moist, helping to avoid infection;
- controlling body temperature by perspiration;
- maintaining brain function.

Water makes up more than half of body weight. Fluid is lost through the urine, faeces, perspiration and breathing, and these losses increase in warmer weather and when a person is physically active, or if they have a fever. Vomiting and diarrhoea can also lead to rapid water loss and this can easily result in dehydration. When a person is dehydrated they can become

130

confused, be susceptible to urinary tract infections, experience headaches, become irritable and be at greater risk of developing pressure sores.

The recommended daily intake of fluid is 1.5–2 litres per day. Most drinks such as juices, milk, tea and coffee in moderation and low-sugar drinks are counted as fluid; however, alcohol can lead to dehydration. Water is the best fluid to rehydrate the body. There are medical conditions, for example some cardiac conditions and some kidney diseases, that require people to drink less fluid. Getting to know the person for whom you are caring or offering support will help you help them: a person's fluid requirements will be detailed in their care plan and you should refer to this when you offer care and support.

Sometimes there will be a requirement for the person not to eat or drink anything for a period of time; this is for their safety, for example before an investigation or an operation. If this is the case ('nil-by-mouth') it will be made clear in the person's care plan.

If dehydration persists and is left untreated, it can have a number of serious consequences. Blood circulation can become compromised and the kidneys can become damaged, which can be a threat to a person's life.

Poor hydration and nutrition

Malnourishment means that a person's diet does not contain the right balance of nutrients required for the person to function effectively. This might include undernutrition, when a person does not get sufficient nutrients, or it could be related to overnutrition, when a person has more nutrients than their body needs. Malnutrition is a condition that is caused by an imbalance between what a person eats and what they need to sustain their health. Malnutrition can result in ill health and can be a consequence of ill health.

Those who provide care or offer people support in the hospital or community setting should do all they can to help people avoid malnutrition. Everyone has a role in making this happen. There are many reasons why people can become malnourished:

- Difficulty eating and swallowing due to ill-fitting dentures or illnesses such as throat cancer; swallowing difficulties due to muscle weakness.
- An inability to absorb nutrients (malabsorption) could be due to nausea and vomiting or diarrhoea or constipation; some medications can also cause this.
- Depression or isolation and loneliness.
- Reduction of taste sensitivity as people get older which can make eating less pleasurable.
- The environment in which the person is eating may cause them to feel uncomfortable.
- A need for increased nutrients.

By understanding more about nutrition, the signs and symptoms of malnutrition and dehydration, and knowing what types of food and drink the people you care for like, you can encourage them to eat and drink the right things. This will help them stay well or get better if they are ill. Signs and symptoms and consequences of malnutrition are outlined in Table 10.2.

The signs and symptoms listed in Table 10.2 may not always be obvious; for example, sometimes weight loss is not obvious because it occurs slowly, over time. You or the person for whom you are caring or offering support might notice that clothing, belts and jewellery gradually feel looser. A person can be overweight or obese and still be malnourished. This may be due to having a diet that consists of food and drink that are high in fat and sugar but low in essential vitamins and minerals.

Figure 10.4 is a urine colour chart that can help to determine if the people you care for or offer support to are hydrated. The chart provides guidelines only with regards to the colour of urine.

Table 10.2   Some signs, symptoms and consequences of malnutrition

Early
Feelings of thirst Dry mouth Passing small amounts of dark, concentrated urine

Later
Weight loss Weight gain Reduced wound healing Headache Apathy and depression Constipation Urinary tract infection Formation of kidney stones Lethargy and sluggishness Vitamin deficiency Impaired immune function (increased risk of infection) Increased risk of pressure sores Muscle wasting and weakness Bone and joint pain Difficulty in keeping warm Impaired respiratory/cardiac function and mobility Poor denture fit Behaviour changes Changes in skin (dryness and rashes) Changes in hair Poor night-time vision Swelling of the tongue, sore mouth, bleeding, swollen gums

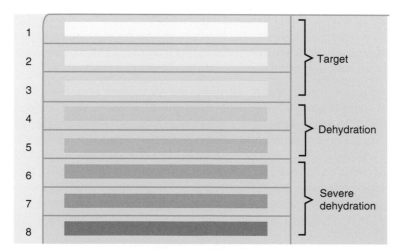

Figure 10.4   Urine colour chart.

Helping people with their nutrition and hydration

Assessment of needs is a key aspect of care provision and this includes an assessment of nutrition and hydration. There are assessment tools available that may help to make an objective assessment of nutritional needs. Elements of assessment will include determining if the person has any food allergies, their preferences (likes and dislikes), and the support they will need to eat and drink. Other information gathered during assessment should determine if the person has their own teeth and, if they do not, whether they can eat normally or require soft food.

133

 ## Stop, look, respond 10.4

Malnutrition Universal Screening Tool

Take some time to look at the national screening tool, the Malnutrition Universal Screening Tool (MUST), which is used to screen people when they are admitted to hospital or a residential care setting.
   Make notes about its use:

_____

_____

_____

_____

_____

Those at high risk of malnutrition can include those people:

- with reduced mobility that can impact on their ability to shop/cook;
- who are housebound;
- living alone;
- who are showing symptoms of depression;
- with dementia;
- who are recovering from serious illness or a condition that is likely to affect their ability to eat, such as a stroke;
- with dental and mouth problems;
- who have a visual impairment;
- who are taking medication whose side effects may affect appetite or cause sickness.

 ## Stop, look, respond 10.5

Visual impairment

How would you promote adequate nutrition and hydration in a person with visual impairment who needs assistance in maintaining their independence when preparing food, eating and drinking?

When providing food for people that is suitable for them and meets their individual needs you must work in a person-centred way. You must consider the person from an individual perspective; consider if the person needs help to open food or drink packets, assistance with cutting up food or holding containers with hot fluids in them.

Determine if the person has any beliefs or preferences that affect the foods that they eat, and ensure these are taken into account. Are there any foods that the person should not have? Some foods may be contraindicated due to their medication; for example some people who are taking certain medications for depression should not eat cheese as this is contraindicated. Vegetarians or vegans choose not to eat certain foods, so it is important that you know what this means.

Stop, look, respond 10.6

Vegans and vegetarians

Make a list of foods that vegans and vegetarians may choose not to eat.

Vegans	Vegetarians

People with specific health conditions should not have certain foods as a result of their health conditions. For example:

- People with high levels of blood cholesterol may be recommended not to have too much saturated fat such as butter, fried items and pastry.
- People with diabetes may be advised to avoid too much sugar, found in sweets, chocolate, sugared breakfast cereals, cakes and puddings, and encouraged to eat fewer of these or eat them in smaller portions.
- People with high blood pressure may be advised to limit salt intake.
- People who are obese should be encouraged to limit their intake of sugary and fatty foods.

Treating people with dignity and respect extends to providing them with appropriate nutrition. You should provide the people for whom you provide care or offer support with enough time to eat; mealtimes should not be rushed and they should be able to choose whether they would like to use any equipment offered (Table 10.3) that can help the person maintain their independence.

You should raise any concerns you may have about a person you are caring for or supporting if they are not eating or drinking enough in spite of you encouraging and supporting them. Expert advice may need to come from a specialist such as a dietician or a nutritionist. An occupational therapist can provide advice about supplementary equipment that can help people maintain their independence.

You may be required to implement closer monitoring of the person's nutrition and fluid intake. Discussing with and observing the person can help to identify any barriers there may be to

Table 10.3   Some equipment available to support people in eating and drinking independently

- Reminders to prompt someone when it is time for them to eat or drink
- Cutlery with padded handles and shaped so as to help with gripping
- Two-handled mugs to help those with a poor grip, tremors or weak wrists
- Cups with lids that can help to reduce the risk of spillage
- One-way straws that help people to drink without the need to lift cups and glasses, even if they have a muscle weakness that has reduced their ability to suck
- Non-slip mats, stopping plates from moving around whilst people are cutting their food
- Plates and bowls with high sides that prevent food falling off the edges
- Insulated bowls to keep the food hot if the person needs more time to eat

eating and drinking. Emphasise that good nutrition and hydration are important in maintaining health and wellbeing. Raise any problems with the person's carer or family member, and consult with other workers such as doctors, therapists or dentists (ensure that the person gives you permission to do this).

Refer to the person's care plan in order to determine individual needs and ensure there is ongoing assessment of nutritional and hydration status. There should be a record in the person's care plan of what the person is eating and drinking and a description of any interventions put in place to prevent malnutrition.

Thinking cap 10.2

Improving mealtimes

Think about the people to whom you offer support or provide care, and consider ways in which you could help to improve mealtimes.

Unless contraindicated or restricted for medical purposes, people should have access to fluids at all times. The healthcare and support worker should encourage the person to drink throughout the day; you should not wait until the person feels thirsty; thirst is an early sign of dehydration. In ensuring that people are drinking adequate amounts you should offer drinks and encourage and support them to drink as described in their care plan. Refresh drinks regularly and place them within easy reach, particularly for people with limited movement or mobility.

The provision of food should be in accordance with the person's care plan; you must ensure that cultural preference and any health conditions and allergen advice are adhered to. There are several food safety principles that will need to be in place when storing, preparing and handling food. If the person's care plan says that they need to be given encouragement to eat, or that they need to be provided with help and support with eating, then you must provide this. Provide food at the right temperature and ensure that it is within easy reach of the person. There may be a need to provide the person with certain types of implements or utensils that will enable them to eat independently; be sure that you provide these.

Stop, look, respond 10.7

Eating and drinking

Make a list and describe ten things that you can do to encourage people who need to eat and drink more.

	Issue	Description
1.		
2.		
3.		
4.		
5.		
6.		
7.		
8.		
9.		
10.		

You must report to a senior member of staff, the person's carer or their family any concerns that you might have about a person's fluid intake, their food or nutrition. You should not delay this as it can lead to dehydration and malnutrition.

Chapter summary

- Mealtimes are more than just about the food that is eaten, it is about who you eat your meals with, what you are eating and how comfortable the environment is.
- It is unacceptable in contemporary society that any person should suffer malnutrition.
- Food safety is essential if people are to be protected from harm.
- There are laws in place that dictate the standards required when storing, preparing and serving food and drinks.
- People can become ill through contaminated food.
- Some people need help and support to access appropriate nutrition.
- Some people in society are more vulnerable than others with regards to food-related illness.
- A range of basic principles must be implemented in order to protect all individuals when handling, storing or preparing food.
- Food and drink offered to people must provide the nutrients required for the body to function effectively.
- Without sufficient fluid the body cannot carry out fundamental processes that will allow it to function effectively.
- Fluid is essential for life.
- There are a range of signs and symptoms that you need to be aware of and that provide the health and care worker with important clues that an individual may be experiencing malnutrition.

- It is essential to undertake a detailed nutritional assessment of nutritional needs using the national assessment tool.
- You should treat people with dignity and respect, providing them with sufficient time to eat. People should not be rushed, and should be able to choose if they would like to use any equipment offered or not.
- The individual's care plan is an essential part of recording and delivering person-centred care.

Case scenario 10.1

Peter

Peter has prostate cancer; he has been admitted to hospital because he is losing weight and he appears to be dehydrated. Peter is 62 years of age, weighs 57 kilograms and is 1.8 metres tall. Using this formula calculate his body mass index (BMI):

$$BMI = weight\ divided\ by\ height\ divided\ by\ height$$
$$(57\ divided\ by\ 1.8\ divided\ by\ 1.8 = BMI)$$

According to the chart below is Peter classified as:

- Underweight?
- Healthy weight?
- Overweight?
- Obese?

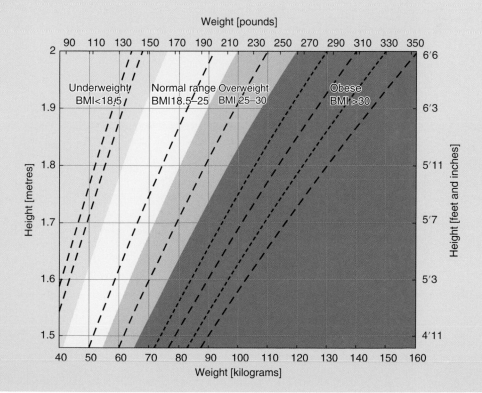

The average amount of water that a person needs to drink every day is 30 millilitres per kilogram of body weight. Peter's body weight is 57 kilograms. Using this formula:

$$\frac{\text{Millilitres multiplied by kilograms}}{(30\text{ multiplied by }57 = \text{amount of fluid per day})}$$

what would be the average amount of water that Peter would need per day?
    In Peter's case how would you promote adequate nutrition and hydration?

 Resource file

The Food Standards Agency
A government site concerned with food safety.
http://www.food.gov.uk

British Association for Parenteral and Enteral Nutrition
A multidisciplinary charity with a membership of doctors, nurses, dieticians, pharmacists, patients and all interested in nutritional care.
http://www.bapen.org.uk

Chapter 11

Awareness of mental health, dementia and learning disability

Care certificate outcomes

1. Understand the needs and experiences of people with mental health conditions, dementia or learning disabilities.
2. Understand the importance of promoting positive health and wellbeing for an individual who may have a mental health condition, dementia or learning disability.
3. Understand the adjustments that may be necessary in care delivery relating to an individual who may have a mental health condition, dementia or learning disability.
4. Understand the importance of early detection of mental health conditions, dementia and learning disabilities.
5. Understand legal frameworks, policy and guidelines relating to mental health conditions, dementia and learning disabilities.
6. Understand the meaning of mental capacity in relation to how care is provided.

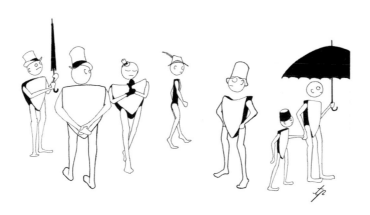

Fundamentals of Care: A Textbook for Health and Social Care Assistants, First Edition. Ian Peate.
© 2017 John Wiley & Sons Ltd. Published 2017 by John Wiley & Sons Ltd.

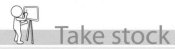

Take stock

Rate your current knowledge and skills prior to reading this chapter. Put a tick in the box that you think applies to you with regards to the standard being discussed:

Key:
I know this I have a good level of knowledge or skills regarding this aspect of the standard. I make use of the knowledge and skills identified on a regular basis, feeling confident in my ability and performance. I do not need a refresher.
Satisfactory My level of knowledge and standard of skills meet the criteria associated with the standard. I use the skills and knowledge from time to time. I might not always feel confident in my capability. I would benefit from a refresher.
I require a review I do not feel that I have the skills and/or the knowledge that would enable me to meet the standard in a confident and competent way. The knowledge and skills I used to have are no longer valid. I will require a refresher.
This is new to me I have never worked in a caring role before or I have never covered this topic before. I will need further training and development in this area.

Standard	Self-assessment			
Understand the needs and experiences of those people with mental health conditions, dementia or learning disabilities	☐ I know this	☐ Satisfactory	☐ I should review this	☐ This is new to me
Explain the value of advancing positive health and wellbeing for those who may have a mental health condition, dementia or learning disability	☐ I know this	☐ Satisfactory	☐ I should review this	☐ This is new to me
Describe adjustments that may be needed in care delivery relating to a person who may have a mental health condition, dementia or learning disability	☐ I know this	☐ Satisfactory	☐ I should review this	☐ This is new to me
Explain the importance of early detection of mental health conditions, dementia and learning disabilities	☐ I know this	☐ Satisfactory	☐ I should review this	☐ This is new to me
Discuss legal frameworks, policy and guidelines associated with mental health conditions, dementia and learning disabilities	☐ I know this	☐ Satisfactory	☐ I should review this	☐ This is new to me
Discuss mental capacity in relation to care provision	☐ I know this	☐ Satisfactory	☐ I should review this	☐ This is new to me

Introduction

Regardless of the area of healthcare or social care in which you work you will meet and may be required to give care or offer support to people with mental health problems, dementia or learning disability. Consequently you will be required to demonstrate awareness and understanding of the care required for this group of people so that any signs and symptoms that concern you are referred to other workers.

People with mental health conditions, dementia or a learning disability will have unique needs. The care or social worker will be required to consider the person from a physical, psychological and social perspective.

Stop, look, respond 11.1

Physical, social, psychological

People who have mental health needs, dementia or learning disabilities face a number of issues, which may be physical, social or psychological and can impact on the person in a number of ways.

Complete the table below to consider the needs and experiences of those with mental health conditions, dementia and learning disabilities, and how these may impact on them physically, socially and psychologically.

	Anxiety	Depression	Dementia	Learning disability
Physically				
Socially				
Psychologically				

It is important to have an understanding of the causes of conditions that may affect this group of people, and as such you will be able to respond and support them with regards to their needs. Needs are different for those with mental health conditions, dementia and learning disabilities.

Mental health conditions

Mental health is everybody's business: individuals, families, employers, educators and communities all need to play their part. Good mental health and resilience are central to physical health, relationships, training, education and work, and in realising aspirations. Mental health problems may not be recognised or acknowledged, and consequently such problems may go untreated and can accelerate in seriousness. This may have a negative impact on the quality of a person's life or it could lead to a deterioration of their mental and physical condition, which may compromise their health and safety. Mental health problems can persist if untreated.

Mental health is difficult to define. It is more than the absence of a mental disorder; it is more about wellbeing, personal contentment and meaning. Mental health can be considered in a positive light, which can identify a positive state of mental wellbeing; or in a negative manner, to identify a negative state of mental wellbeing.

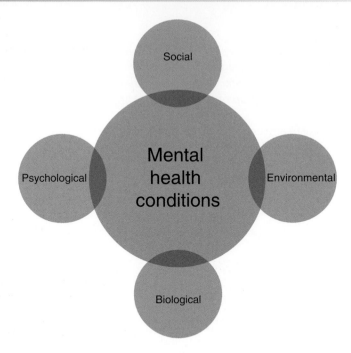

Figure 11.1   Mental health conditions and interrelationships.

A mental illness is a condition that impacts a person's thinking, feeling or mood and can affect the individual's ability to relate to others and to function on a daily basis. It affects a person's ability to make the most of opportunities that arise and to play a full part with their family, when at work, in the community and with their friends.

Each person will have different experiences, even those people with the same diagnosis. There are many different mental health conditions that people can develop; they include:

- psychosis;
- depression;
- anxiety.

A mental health condition is not the result of one event, but of multiple, interlinking causes. The causes of mental health problems are not known; it is most probable that social, psychological, biological and environmental factors interact in a number of ways that increase the risk of a person developing a mental disorder (Figure 11.1).

People with mental health conditions, dementia and learning disabilities are dissimilar groups encompassing people with a very diverse range of needs and preferences. Service providers therefore are required to deliver a personalised approach that is built around the needs of the individual person.

Mental health influences and is influenced by a wide and complex range of factors that cut across different spheres of life, for example:

- health (physical and mental);
- employment;
- financial problems;
- housing;

Table 11.1   Mental health statistics

- At some point in their life at least one in four people will experience a mental health problem. At any one time one in six adults has a mental health problem
- One in ten children aged between 5 and 16 years has a mental health problem, and many continue to have mental health problems as they grow into adulthood
- Half of those with lifetime mental health problems first experience symptoms by the age of 14 years, and three-quarters before their mid-20s
- In young people self-harming is not uncommon (10–13% of 15–16-year-olds have self-harmed)
- Around 50% of all adults will experience at least one episode of depression during their lifetime
- One in ten new mothers experience postnatal depression
- Approximately 1 in 100 people has a severe mental health problem
- Around 60% of adults living in hostels have a personality disorder
- Some 90% of all prisoners are estimated to have a diagnosable mental health problem (including personality disorder) and/or a substance misuse problem

- leisure;
- lifestyle;
- social networks;
- bereavement.

These factors and triggers (i.e. bereavement), individually or collectively, can impact on whether a person develops a mental health condition. A multi-agency approach is required to address needs in a holistic way.

Stress or a challenging home life can make some people more vulnerable to mental health problems. This is also true of traumatic life events, for example being the victim of a crime. Biochemical processes and other biological activity may play a role in the development and the recovery from a mental health condition.

Many people experience a mental health problem at some point in their lives. It has been predicted that at any given time, one in six adults has a mental health problem of varying severity. Problems can range from mild depression and anxiety through to psychosis and severe personality disorders. The person's problems may be temporary or they could be long term; they may fluctuate in incidence and severity during the course of a person's lifetime. Table 11.1 provides an overview of a range of mental health statistics.

There are strong links between mental health conditions and social exclusion; the prevalence of mental ill health is not evenly distributed across the country. Those with mental health problems often have fewer educational qualifications, find it harder to get work, have lower incomes and live in areas with higher socio-economic deprivation. Associated with this, they are also more likely to experience difficulties in accessing services and receiving a full range of support in response to their needs.

Service provision

In the UK the delivery of mental health care service provision is organised in a three-tier structure:

- primary
- secondary
- tertiary care

Over the years the provision of mental health care has changed. There has been an emphasis on maximising efficiency and reducing costs, whilst providing treatment and offering people support in the least restrictive and socially inclusive way. Most people with a mental health condition are cared for in community settings; only the people who are most acutely unwell and those with complex needs are cared for in hospital settings.

The primary care setting refers to non-specialist care services provided through GP surgeries. Often it is the GP who is the first point of contact for those who are experiencing mental distress. Responses from these professionals will reflect their skills, attitudes and experience.

Secondary care services are specialist mental health services that are based in community settings. The key role of secondary care services is to assess and treat people with acute, severe and/or enduring mental health problems. Specialist services exist for older people with organic mental health problems, including dementia. Prompt and effective treatment has been shown to improve long-term mental health.

Tertiary care mental health services refer to inpatient care, usually provided in hospital-based settings. These acute services are made up of assessment and recovery wards, psychiatric intensive care units and forensic services.

Depression

Depression is a mood disorder, an illness that is characterised by low mood and a wide range of other possible symptoms; these will vary from person to person. Most people experience feelings of sadness, being down, being fed up or being unhappy; however, living with depression is different. We can all go through periods of feeling down, but when a person is depressed they feel persistently sad for weeks or months, as opposed to just a few days. A person who is experiencing depression will feel emotions such as hopelessness and negativity that will not go away.

Some may think that depression is something petty, unimportant and that it is not a genuine health condition. Depression is the most common psychiatric disorder, and it is an illness with real symptoms, not a sign of weakness or something a person can 'get over with' or snap out of by 'pulling themselves together'. With the right treatment and support, the majority of people will be able to make a full recovery. If depression is not treated, however, it can become a chronic (long-standing) illness with ensuing disability.

Depression can develop quickly or it may come on gradually, and be brought on or made worse by life events and/or changes in body chemistry. Depression will not just go away, and it can happen to anyone. Depression refers to both negative affect (low mood) and/or absence of positive affect (loss of interest and pleasure in most activities). As well as this the person may be experiencing a range of emotional, cognitive, physical and behavioural symptoms.

The severity of the condition is based on the extent of symptoms and their functional impact, and ranges from sub-threshold depression to severe depression – in a continuum (Figure 11.2).

The symptoms of depression may endure for one or two weeks, a number of months or even longer. Those people who are living with depression can have problems with how they see themselves, and this can cause them not to engage with others socially, with their family or with their work. Table 11.2 outlines some of the physical symptoms that people may experience.

With the right support and treatment, most people with depression can make a full recovery. Treatments that are available to support those with depression include providing them with the opportunity to talk and share how they are feeling (talking treatments). There are a number of

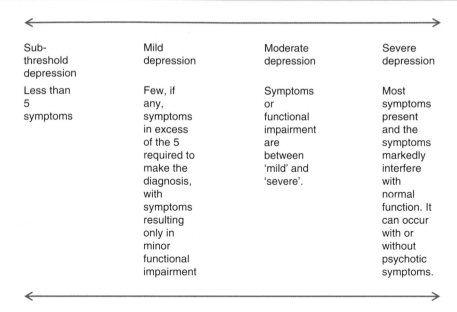

Figure 11.2   Severity of depression on a continuum.

Table 11.2   Some physical symptoms that people with depression may experience

- Feeling constantly tired
- Sleeping badly
- Having no appetite or a change in appetite
- Having no sex drive (loss of libido)
- Experiencing various aches and pains
- Changes in menstrual cycle

Table 11.3   Some treatment options for depression

Mild to moderate depression

- Talking therapy – a type of psychotherapy such as cognitive behavioural therapy and counselling

Moderate to severe depression

- Antidepressants – medication that treats the symptoms of depression
- Combination therapy – a course of antidepressants plus talking therapy
- Mental health teams – the person with severe depression may be referred to a mental health team made up of psychologists, psychiatrists, specialist nurses and occupational therapists. These teams often provide intensive specialist talking treatments as well as prescribed medication

organisations that support individuals who are experiencing depression, and they can provide additional information on the condition. Medication or a combination of medication and talking treatments can be prescribed. The kind of treatment will depend on the type of depression the person has; see Table 11.3.

Anxiety

This is a feeling of unease, worry or fear. We have all felt anxious at some point in our lives, but for some people this can be an ongoing problem. Those who are living with anxiety can find it difficult to control their worries. They may feel that things are worse than they are, and this can result in a number of other symptoms. Symptoms of anxiety can be both psychological and physical. Table 11.4 outlines the psychological (these are symptoms that are related to emotions and feelings), physical and behavioural symptoms that may be associated with anxiety.

Treatments are available that help alleviate the symptoms of anxiety, for example, cognitive behavioural therapy and mindfulness (these are approaches that encourage the person to think about themselves, the world and other people). Talking to people in this way helps the person to talk about their condition and to manage the effects by trying to change the way that they think.

If the psychological treatments have not helped the person or if they would prefer not to try them, then they may be offered medication. Referral may also be made to a mental health specialist.

Table 11.4   Psychological, physical and behavioural symptoms associated with anxiety

Psychological
• Feeling worried or uneasy much of the time • Having difficulty with sleep, causing tiredness • Finding it difficult to concentrate • Being irritable • Being extra alert • Feeling on edge or not being able to relax • Needing and seeking frequent reassurance from other people • Feeling tearful • Thinking negative thoughts

Physical
• A pounding heartbeat • Breathing faster • Palpitations • Feeling sick • Chest pains • Headaches • Sweating • A loss of appetite • Feeling faint • Needing to use the toilet more frequently • Feeling of 'butterflies' in the stomach

Behavioural
• Not wanting to leave the house • Abusing substances such as alcohol or drugs • Behaving in ways that affect relationships • Not going out with friends • Not going out to places such as the supermarket

Bipolar disorder

This condition, which used to be called manic depression, causes the person to experience periods of extreme mood swings, ranging from highs (mania), such as joy and excitement, to feelings of absolute misery and hopelessness (depression). Because of this the person may behave in ways that others find difficult to understand. Some people may experience moods that can last for several weeks (or even longer), and some may not experience a 'normal' mood very often.

Psychosis

This is a symptom of conditions such as schizophrenia and bipolar disorder. Schizophrenia (a lifelong condition) is the most common form of psychosis; the condition can be either a chronic form or a form with relapsing and remitting episodes of acute illness.

Schizophrenia is a serious mental health condition that causes disordered ideas, beliefs and experiences, and the cause is unclear. In many ways those with schizophrenia can lose touch with reality and do not know which thoughts and experiences are true and real and which are not. Symptoms may include:

- hallucinations (a person sees or hears things that are not real but to them are very real; this may also include feeling, smelling or tasting things that are not real);
- delusions (where a person believes things that are not true, e.g. believing that someone is listening in on their telephone calls);
- disordered thoughts;
- changes in behaviour;
- problems with motivation;
- emotions may become flat.

In many people symptoms come back (recur) or persist long-term but some people have just one episode of symptoms that lasts a few weeks. Schizophrenia affects not only the person but also their family and close friends. When a person experiences a psychotic event this can be frightening and may cause them to behave in ways that others might think strange.

Offering support to a person who is experiencing an hallucination or delusion is to let them know that you are there to help them and that they are safe as opposed to telling them that you cannot see or hear what they think they are seeing or hearing. This approach prevents them from feeling that you do not believe them; this might help to relieve their stress.

Most people who experience psychosis will, with the use of medication and the provision of social support, get better. In some cases, however, the person may have to be admitted to hospital for treatment and support. If this is the case the person's individual needs will need to be assessed and a plan of care formulated.

Dementia

Dementia is not a single illness; it describes a group of symptoms that have been caused by damage to the brain. Changes associated with dementia are often small to start with, but for a person with dementia they have become severe enough to affect their daily life.

Dementia is not an unavoidable consequence of getting older and is not associated with any particular ethnic group, gender or culture; people from all walks of life may be affected. The condition is progressive, which means that the symptoms will gradually get worse. The speed at which dementia progresses depends on the individual person and the type of dementia that they have. Each person is unique and will experience dementia in their own

Table 11.5   Some symptoms associated with dementia

- Short-term memory loss, such as remembering past events much more easily than recent ones or finding it hard to follow conversations or TV programmes
- Problems in thinking
- Problems with reasoning and problem-solving
- Feeling anxious, depressed or angry about memory loss
- Feeling confused, even when in a familiar environment

way, but in the later stages the person will have problems undertaking everyday tasks and caring for themselves.

A person with dementia may also experience changes in their mood or behaviour. The specific symptoms a person with dementia experiences will depend on the parts of the brain that are damaged and the disease causing the dementia. See Table 11.5 for the symptoms associated with dementia.

Making a diagnosis of dementia can be difficult, and a number of investigations are needed, for example:

- the Mini Mental State Examination;
- CT scan;
- a detailed personal history.

Making a diagnosis can help a person to make decisions about life events, plan for their future, and make advance statements and/or advanced directives; it also helps in the provision of appropriate medications. If a person's dementia is associated with a genetic component then this information can be of value to other family members. Advance statements ensure that the person's wishes are taken into account in the future, often referred to as advance care planning. The aim is to enable the individual to make choices and decisions about their future care. This can ensure that the person is not given any care or treatment that they do not want to receive but that they will receive the care they wish to have.

Stop, look, respond 11.2

What is the Mini Mental State Examination?

_____
_____
_____
_____
_____

Dementia is caused by a number of diseases of the brain, of which Alzheimer's disease is the most common. The second most common cause is vascular dementia. High blood pressure, heart problems, high cholesterol and diabetes may increase the chances of developing vascular dementia. It is important therefore that these conditions are identified and treated at the earliest opportunity. Table 11.6 describes the two most common causes of dementia.

Table 11.6 Two most common causes of dementia

Alzheimer's disease

Alzheimer's disease kills brain cells and nerves; this results in changes in the chemistry and the structure of the brain. As the number of nerves reduces then the brain shrinks in size. Neurotransmitters (chemicals in the brain) are reduced and levels of a particular chemical, acetylcholine, falls. Then gaps develop in the temporal lobe of the brain and other structures; these structures are responsible for the storage and retrieval information

There are lapses of memory and problems finding the right words; there may be mood swings; the person can become withdrawn. They experience difficulty in carrying out everyday tasks

Vascular dementia (multiple infarct dementia)

This is caused by oxygen failing to reach the brain cells due to problems with the blood supply (the vascular system). This results in infarcts (strokes) that occur within the small blood vessels of the brain; these are so small that they go unrecognised. As oxygen supply to the brain is diminished then brain cells die

After each infarct, brain tissue also dies, leaving the person unable to manage daily activities; eventually the person will become confused and unable to cope. There are often problems with the speed of thinking, concentration and communication, and the person may be depressed and experience anxiety. Symptoms of stroke, such as physical weakness or paralysis, can be apparent

A person who experiences problems associated with dementia may feel confused, frustrated and frightened. Short-term memory loss (a common symptom) can mean that the person finds it difficult to remember recent events or conversations. This may mean that they will repeat stories or may ask the same question over and over again.

 ## Thinking cap 11.1

People with dementia

Each person will respond differently to the difficulties that they may experience with regards to dementia. Dementia can have an effect on a person's feelings and emotions.

Think about the various feelings and emotions that may arise in a person with dementia who is experiencing memory problems.

As dementia is a progressive condition the health or social care worker may be supporting people at all stages of their journey. Whilst you are required to provide care to the individual you may also be required to support the person's family.

 ## Stop, look, respond 11.3

Types of dementia

As well as Alzheimer's disease and vascular dementia there are other types of dementia, such as:

- Lewy body
- Korsakoff syndrome
- Parkinson's disease
- Creutzfeldt–Jakob disease
- Huntington's disease

Choose one of the above and learn more about it and record your findings.

Learning disabilities

The experience for a person living with a learning disability will vary and this will also be true for the person offering care or support to that person and their family.

As with other people to whom you offer care or support, those with a learning disability are unique individuals who have their own likes and dislikes, who express their own opinions, and have their own history. They have the same rights as anyone else and as such should not be excluded or discriminated against. Learning disability is a common, lifelong condition; it is neither an illness nor a disease. Learning disability is used in relation to individuals who have a significant impairment of intelligence and/or a significant impairment of adaptive functioning; usually onset occurs prior to adulthood (in the developmental period). It is the learning disability that is defined not the person; your focus should be on people who have a learning disability as opposed to a specific learning difficulty. People with learning disability have a wide and diverse range of needs and preferences; they are a mixed group.

Sometimes there is confusion between learning disabilities and mental health problems. Having a learning disability is not the same as having a mental health problem, such as depression or anxiety. However, anyone can be affected by mental health problems, including those with learning disabilities. All health and social care workers have a role in promoting the mental health of people with learning disabilities.

Stop, look, respond 11.4

Definitions

Other countries use differing terms. For example, in Ireland, the USA and Canada they use the term 'intellectual disability' for what we would describe as a learning disability.

The Department of Health uses the term 'learning disability' within their policy and practice documents. The Department of Health provides a definition in 'Valuing People' (Department of Health (2001) Valuing People: A New Strategy for Learning Disability for the 21st Century. London: DH.)

Access this document and find out how they describe a 'learning disability'.

Learning disability is a result of brain development being affected before birth (in utero), during the birth of the child or in a person's childhood. A person with learning disability may have difficulty understanding information, learning new skills, communicating, carrying out everyday tasks and living their lives independently.

Degree of learning disability

If you are caring for or offering support to a person with learning disability, you may come across one of the following descriptions of degree of learning disability:

- mild
- moderate
- severe
- profound

Table 11.7   Degrees of learning disability

Degree	Description
Mild	Most people with learning disabilities have mild learning disabilities. The majority of these people live independently; they have their own families, they are employed and do not require extra support from services, unless in crisis
Moderate	For those with a moderate learning disability, the level of support required is higher. Many will need some level of support with everyday tasks and they might have difficulty in communicating their needs. It is likely that they will be living with their parents, with day-to-day support, or living in supported living schemes. People with moderate learning disability are also likely to use a number of support services, e.g. day centres, outreach and supported living arrangements
Severe/profound	People who have a severe and profound learning disability may have considerably increased health needs, e.g. greater rates of epilepsy, sensory impairments and physical disabilities. These people usually have more complex needs and can experience greater difficulty when communicating their needs. In an effort to communicate their needs or as a way of expressing their frustration some people engage in behaviour that others consider challenging. In some people with a profound learning disability self-injury is common, and this may lead to additional disability, poor health and a significantly diminished quality of life People with a severe and profound learning disability can also be described as people who have high support needs

These descriptions come originally from a medical perspective. Policy makers are now encouraging services to focus on service provision that emphasises an individual's needs as opposed to the grouping together of people with learning disabilities. These terms, however, are still commonly used. Table 11.7 provides broad descriptions.

The categories listed in Table 11.7 appear to be distinct categories. However, these do not adequately describe the range of ability/impairment/disability that people with a learning disability may have. These are generalised categories, and some people with a learning disability will overlap them.

A person with autism, for example, who has learning disabilities, could have substantial social difficulties and appear to have moderate learning difficulties. However, they may be able to look after their own personal care and everyday needs independently.

Thinking cap 11.2

People with a learning difficulty

Think of a time when you have observed a person with a learning disability respond in a way that others (maybe yourself) have found challenging/disturbing.
   How did those observing this person react?

Causes of learning disabilities

The causes of a learning disability may not always be known. Some learning disabilities are the result of genetics; Down syndrome, for example, is due to an extra chromosome. Down syndrome can lead to impairments in the person's cognitive ability and their physical growth, which can range from mild to moderate developmental disabilities. Other causes include complications during the birth of the child leading to a lack of oxygen, or the child may be born prematurely. Illness or injury in childhood that has affected the brain such as meningitis or other childhood illnesses can also lead to a learning disability.

It may not always be obvious that a person has a learning disability. In some cases the person shows specific physical characteristics, for example, those caused by Down syndrome. However, this is not always the case. Understanding the cause of a person's learning disability and recognising someone's learning disabilities quickly, may mean that you can respond more appropriately to their needs and if required you can seek the advice of specialist learning disability professionals.

In many instances living with a learning disability will have a lifelong impact on the person and their family, but this can vary depending on the type of learning disability the person has.

Providing care and support

In order to deliver and provide services that are of a high quality a personalised approach is required, one that is built around the needs of the individual. Any approach to service provision involves multiple agencies working together to deliver a person-centred approach, one that listens, learns and focuses on what is important to the person, working with others to act on this and make things happen.

Those with learning disabilities are significantly more likely to have health problems than other people. Despite this people with learning disabilities have higher levels of unmet needs and receive less effective treatment, even though the law explicitly sets out a legal framework for the delivery of equal treatment. Life expectancy is increasing in people with mild learning disabilities, and is approaching that of the general population. But mortality rates among people with moderate to severe learning disabilities are three times higher than in the general population. Despite this people with learning disabilities have a shorter life expectancy when compared to those in the general population.

Discrimination, inequality and exclusion are prominent in those with a learning disability, and such people are often stigmatised. Stigma can have a negative impact on a person's self-esteem and self-image, and with stigma comes unemployment and social isolation. Stigma often results from misconceptions about people with a learning disability; it can be seen as a mark of shame or discredit, a sign of social unacceptability. Figure 11.3 considers the cycle of stigma.

A label is applied to a group that distinguishes them from others, and the label is assigned to undesirable attributes of the group (deviance). People with the label are seen as different from those without the label, thus contributing to an 'us' versus 'them' outlook, and those with the label are unfairly discriminated against.

Stigma is often linked to living with a mental health need, dementia or learning disability and the outcome can result in feelings of loneliness or being left out of society (exclusion). Focusing on the person's abilities and skills and fostering a positive attitude can help to begin to address these negative issues and the person can be supported to live well:

- Ensure that people are not isolated in social situations.
- Promote wellbeing for those who are living with the condition.
- Identify and build on the skills and abilities the person has.
- Provide opportunities for people to feel empowered and to be in control.

The social model of disability

The social model of disability has at its core the notion that disability is caused by the way society is organised, as opposed to a person's impairment or difference. It considers the ways of removing barriers that restrict life choices for people with a disability. The model points out

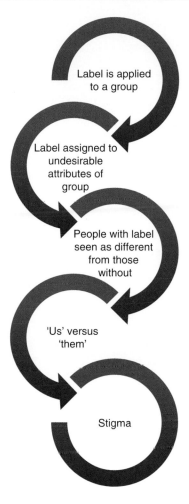

Figure 11.3   The cycle of stigma.

Table 11.8   Some barriers that can prevent people with a disability from living independently

- Insufficient funding of services
- Physical barriers in the built environment, e.g. a building that is inaccessible for wheelchair users
- Failure to make reasonable adjustments to services so that they can be easily and effectively used by service users
- Negative attitudes and values from staff. Staff making assumptions and stereotyping
- Lack of staff training
- Inflexible organisational procedures, where organisational procedures are set to meet the needs of the organisation as opposed to the individual
- Inaccessible information – presented in a format that the person cannot understand and use
- Inability to access healthcare facilities, e.g. screening programmes
- Lack of support services
- Failure to offer choice and encourage participation

that when barriers are removed, disabled people can be independent and equal in society and will have choice and control over their own lives. See Table 11.8 for some barriers that can prevent people with a disability from making choices or living independently.

Stop, look, respond 11.5

Values and attitudes

We all have different values and attitudes. What one person values may differ from that of another person. A person's attitudes are revealed in how they respond to situations or people.

Make a list of five things that you value:

1.
2.
3.
4.
5.

Thinking of these values, how did you get them?

What do you think influenced your values?

How easy do you think it would be to change those values that you hold?

The implementation of the social model of disability ensures that the focus is on the individual and their individual needs and not on the person's condition. Disabled people developed the social model of disability. This was because the traditional model of care, the medical model, was unable to explain the disabled person's own experience of disability nor was it able to develop more inclusive ways of living. This model can help to develop positive attitudes in society.

Stop, look, respond 11.6

The medical model of disability

The social model of disability says that a disability is caused by the way society is organised, rather than by a person's impairment or difference. The medical model of disability focuses on treating or trying to cure an illness. Under the medical model it would be suggested that impairments or differences should be and can be fixed or changed by medical and other treatments, even when the impairment or difference does not cause the person pain or illness.

Write notes about why you think the medical model is an inappropriate model to use when caring for or offering support to people with disability.

_____

_____

_____

_____

_____

_____

Assessing and making a diagnosis

An early diagnosis of a mental health problem or dementia will benefit the individual, their family and their friends. Support mechanisms can be put in place to maximise the person's quality of life. The diagnosis will help to clear up any doubt or uncertainties about a person's health and wellbeing, and this may help the person and family understand what and why some things, such as changes in memory and personality, are occurring. Many conditions can have similar symptoms and because of this it is important that an accurate diagnosis is made.

When a definitive diagnosis is made this can also help the person feel more in control, enabling the person and their family and friends to make plans. When this occurs it can provide the opportunity to consider, discuss and record any individual wishes and decisions.

Advance care planning occurs when the individual makes plans about what they wish to happen to them while they are most able to be involved and make decisions. An early diagnosis can provide the opportunity to identify potential treatments and therapies that may be available; for example, the individual may wish to think about taking anti-dementia drugs or antidepressant medications. The person might also benefit from therapies such as counselling or cognitive behaviour therapy (talking therapies). Accessing information (this has to be accurate and easily accessible) at an early stage enables the person to make best use of what is available, such as support groups.

Living with a mental health need, dementia or learning disability may mean that there could be a requirement to change how care and support is offered over time. This will ensure that care and support remains person-centred, adapting to and responding to the individual's needs. Changes could mean that the health and care worker may be required to develop skills to support people who find it a challenge to communicate verbally, for example, learning British Sign Language or Makaton. Assistive technology such as clocks and calendars, reminder messages, interactive message boards or locator devices may be required, and the worker will need to learn how to use this technology as is the case with the person himself or herself.

Mental capacity

A number of polices and pieces of legislation are in place to promote human rights, inclusion, equal life chances and citizenship of those with mental health needs, dementia or learning disabilities (Table 11.9).

The term 'mental capacity' means that a person is able to make his or her own decisions; the person is able to understand information and make an informed decision or choice.

Table 11.9   Legal frameworks and policy and guidance

Legislation/policy	Description
Human Rights Act 1998	This sets out the fundamental rights and freedoms that all people have access to in the UK. The Act protects all of us, rich and poor, old and young. The Act ensures that those with mental health needs, dementia or learning disabilities are also treated fairly and with respect
Care Act 2014	The Care Act is primarily for adults who are in need of care and support and their adult carers. This puts a general duty on local authorities to promote the wellbeing of individuals The Act outlines the way in which local authorities should carry out carers' assessments and needs assessments; how local authorities should determine who is eligible for support; the new obligations on local authorities; and how local authorities should charge for both residential care and community care. The emphasis is on prevention and ensuring that things do not get worse for a person; providing information to ensure people can make informed decisions; and ensuring there are a range of services available to meet the needs of people
Data Protection Act 1998	This ensures that public bodies maintain the protection of data. The Data Protection Act ensures that personal data held by organisations is kept confidential, is not retained longer than needed and is accurate. The data held may be about a person's health or condition. The Act provides people with the right to see the data and information held about them
The Equality Act 2010	This Act legally protects people from discrimination in the workplace and in wider society. It replaced previous anti-discrimination laws with a single Act, making the law easier to understand and strengthening protection in some situations
Safeguarding Adults National Framework	The promotion of people's welfare and keeping them safe from harm and abuse is the core of this framework, which is concerned with safeguarding
Fundamental Standards of Quality and Safety	This is a guide that has been developed by the Care Quality Commission and describes the fundamental standards of quality and safety that those people using health and social care services can expect The fundamental standards define the basic standards of safety and quality that should always be met

A person who lacks capacity as a result of an illness or disability, for example a mental health problem, dementia or a learning disability, cannot do one or more of the following four things:

1. Understand information given to them about a particular decision.
2. Retain that information long enough to be able to make the decision.
3. Weigh up the information available to make the decision.
4. Communicate their decision.

All people have the right to make their own decisions. We all make decisions, big and small, every day of our lives. Most of us are able to make these decisions for ourselves, although we may seek information, advice or support for those more serious or complicated decisions that we make.

Thinking cap 11.3

Making decisions

Think about those large and small decisions that you have made. What decisions did you make without any help from anyone else and what decisions did you make that required you to seek help from others?

For some people their capacity to make certain decisions about their life can be affected temporarily or permanently. A person with a learning disability, for example, might lack the capacity to make major decisions; this does not necessarily mean, however, that the person cannot decide what to eat, or what to wear and do each day. A person who has mental health problems may be unable to make decisions when they are unwell, but able to make them when they are well. A person with dementia is likely to lose the ability to make decisions as the dementia gets more severe.

Assuming that a person has capacity means that opportunities can be provided that can allow the person to make their own decisions, which will help them to feel empowered, confident and in control.

Assessing capacity

A mental capacity assessment is decision-specific; the principles have to be applied to individual decisions. An individual may lack the capacity to make a specific decision, for example regarding their finances, but this does not mean that the person lacks capacity to make all decisions.

The Mental Capacity Act 2005 (this is different from the Mental Health Act) exists to ensure that adults who lack the capacity to make decisions for themselves are protected under the law. This Act applies not only to people with mental health problems, dementia and learning disability but also to those who may have a brain injury or who are under the influence of substances or sedation. The Act assists and supports people who may lack capacity, preventing anyone who is involved in caring for someone who lacks capacity from being overly restrictive or controlling. It also aims to balance a person's right to make decisions for themselves and protecting them from harm if they lack capacity to make decisions to protect themselves.

A person is said to lack capacity if they are unable to:

- understand information relevant to the decision; or
- remember the information for long enough to enable them to make the decision; or
- weigh up information relevant to the decision; or
- communicate their decision – by talking, using sign language, or by any other means such as eye blinking.

See Table 11.10 for the principles to be followed when assessing capacity.

A test of capacity has two stages. Firstly, consideration must be given to whether there is an impairment or disturbance in the functioning of a person's mind or brain. Secondly, if such an impairment exists, is this sufficient to lead to a lack of capacity to make a particular decision?

Table 11.10   Principles to be followed when assessing capacity

- Always assume that the person is able to make their own decision
- Provide all possible support to ensure the person can make their own decision
- Never assume a person is unable to make a decision because you feel they are making an unwise or unsafe decision
- If it has been identified that the person cannot make a decision, it must be deemed to be in that person's best interest before someone else makes a decision on their behalf
- If a decision is made on behalf of the individual, this must be the least restrictive option

Importantly, a person has capacity unless the contrary has been established; people must be helped to make decisions. Unwise decisions do not always mean lack of capacity. Decisions taken on behalf of the person must be in the person's best interests and they must be as least restrictive of freedom as possible.

Stop, look, respond 11.7

Reporting concerns

You often need confidence in sharing a concern that you might have, and you might be concerned as to whether or not sharing this concern is the right thing to do. You may have questions such as: How do I raise a concern? Who should I tell? What should I do if the concern is not addressed in an appropriate way? It is important to act promptly when raising your concerns.

You must be familiar with your organisation's policy on raising concerns. Obtain a copy of your own organisation's agreed procedure that informs you how to report concerns that are related to any unmet needs that can arise from mental health conditions, dementia or learning disability. Think about who you might go to about reporting your concerns.

Chapter summary

- The needs and experiences of those with mental health conditions, dementia or learning disabilities are related to the unique circumstance the person finds themself in.
- People must be cared for on an individual basis.
- The health or social care worker has an important role to play in the promotion of positive health and wellbeing for people who may have a mental health condition, dementia or learning disability.
- Adjustments that are required in care delivery relating to an individual who may have a mental health condition, dementia or learning disability must be made after a holistic assessment of needs has been undertaken.
- Early detection of mental health conditions, dementia and learning disabilities can have a positive impact on the person's health and social outcomes. An early diagnosis can support the person to put steps in place to maximise their quality of life.
- There are a number of legal frameworks, policies and guidelines that relate to mental health conditions, dementia and learning disabilities.

- Those who provide healthcare and offer support to those with mental health conditions, dementia and learning disabilities must have an understanding of the meaning of mental capacity in relation to how care is provided.
- If there is any confusion, misunderstanding or concern regarding the care of those with mental health conditions, dementia and learning disabilities, the person providing care or offering support must raise these concerns and should seek advice and assistance from senior staff.

 ## Case scenario 11.1

Robbie

Robbie is a 23-year-old man who has learning disabilities, epilepsy and autism. He lives in a basement flat and receives three hours outreach support twice a week from a local charitable service.

He has a number of interests including reading books about the prehistoric era and comics, he enjoys train spotting and, when the fair is in town, going to the fair.

Robbie attends computer classes at his local college and for one day a week the local library employs him. He does not have many friends; however, he does enjoy the company of other people.

Robbie finds it hard to understand the subtle rules and social skills that govern interaction, and others often see him as coming across as rude.

How might you help to support Robbie, particularly when it comes to meeting and interacting with other people?

 ## Resource file

Mental Health Foundation
The UK's leading mental health research, policy and service improvement charity.
http://www.mentalhealth.org.uk

Department of Health (2011)
No health without mental health: A cross-government mental health outcomes strategy for people of all ages
https://www.gov.uk/government/uploads/system/uploads/attachment_data/file/213761/dh_124058.pdf

Mencap
This link takes you to the full Death by Indifference report:
http://www.hscbereavementnetwork.hscni.net/wp-content/uploads/2014/05/Death-by-Indifference-Mencap-March-2007.pdf

Chapter 12

Safeguarding adults

Care certificate outcomes

1. Understand the principles of safeguarding adults.
2. Reduce the likelihood of abuse.
3. Respond to suspected or disclosed abuse.
4. Protect people from harm and abuse – locally and nationally.

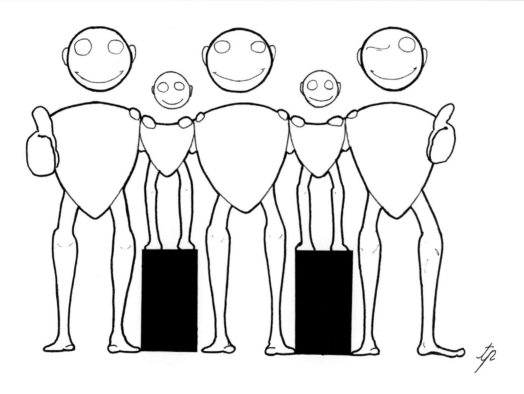

Fundamentals of Care: A Textbook for Health and Social Care Assistants, First Edition. Ian Peate.
© 2017 John Wiley & Sons Ltd. Published 2017 by John Wiley & Sons Ltd.

Take stock

Rate your current knowledge and skills prior to reading this chapter. Put a tick in the box that you think applies to you with regards to the standard being discussed:

Key:
I know this
I have a good level of knowledge or skills regarding this aspect of the standard. I make use of the knowledge and skills identified on a regular basis, feeling confident in my ability and performance. I do not need a refresher.
Satisfactory
My level of knowledge and standard of skills meet the criteria associated with the standard. I use the skills and knowledge from time to time. I might not always feel confident in my capability. I would benefit from a refresher.
I require a review
I do not feel that I have the skills and/or the knowledge that would enable me to meet the standard in a confident and competent way. The knowledge and skills I used to have are no longer valid. I will require a refresher.
This is new to me
I have never worked in a caring role before or I have never covered this topic before. I will need further training and development in this area.

Standard	Self-assessment			
Understand the principles that underpin safeguarding adults	☐ I know this	☐ Satisfactory	☐ I should review this	☐ This is new to me
Discuss your role in reducing the likelihood of abuse	☐ I know this	☐ Satisfactory	☐ I should review this	☐ This is new to me
Describe how you would respond to suspected or disclosed abuse	☐ I know this	☐ Satisfactory	☐ I should review this	☐ This is new to me
Outline how people can be protected from harm and abuse locally and nationally	☐ I know this	☐ Satisfactory	☐ I should review this	☐ This is new to me

Introduction

Safeguarding is everyone's business, and abuse of anyone by anyone is wrong. Yours is an important role in safeguarding adults. Safeguarding adults is one of the key responsibilities of the health or social care worker, which means responding to needs appropriately and protecting people from harm or abuse. Those offering care or support to people need to identify the most common forms of abuse, how to report any suspected cases, and how to act in such a way as to prevent further abuse by reporting and responding effectively to any issues that may be disclosed or suspected.

This chapter explains key terms related to safeguarding adults, such as abuse and harm. The role and responsibilities of those who provide care or offer support with regards to safeguarding individuals are discussed. A range of factors that feature in adult abuse and neglect are outlined, stressing the importance of ensuring that people are treated with dignity and respect when providing services.

The importance of individualised, person-centred care is reiterated, with an emphasis on how to apply the principles of helping people to keep themselves safe. Arrangements for the implementation of multi-agency Safeguarding Adults policies and procedures are described.

Responding to suspected or disclosed abuse is considered, with an explanation of what to do if abuse of an adult is suspected; including how to raise concerns using local policy and procedure. Relevant legislation and local and national policies and procedures concerning safeguarding adults are described along with an explanation of the importance of sharing information with the relevant agencies.

Anyone may find himself or herself in a difficult situation where there is a chance that they could be harmed, but when the situation involves a person who needs extra support then this is known as 'an adult at risk' and the situation becomes serious.

Safeguarding

Safeguarding adults is about protecting those at risk of harm (vulnerable adults) from suffering abuse or neglect. Abuse can happen anywhere – at home, in a residential or nursing home, in a hospital, at work or in the street. Safeguarding vulnerable adults is complex. The group (vulnerable adults) is extremely wide and can range from adults who are incapable of looking after any aspect of their lives, to those who experience a short episode of illness or disability. Some people in our society are more at risk than others.

Stop, look, respond 12.1

Those at greater risk

List some of the things that might lead to someone being at greater risk of abuse:

_____
_____
_____
_____
_____
_____

Protecting people includes offering them support regarding their wellbeing, ensuring that their fundamental needs, for example safety, nutrition and hydration, are met. Safeguarding promotes a person's independence. All adults should be able to live their lives free from fear and harm, should expect to be treated with dignity and respect, and have their rights and choices respected. Safeguarding of adults aims to ensure that each person is able to maintain to the best of their abilities:

- dignity and respect;
- quality of life;

- health;
- choice;
- control;
- safety.

A vulnerable adult is said to be a person who is receiving or may need to receive community care services because of a mental health problem or other disability, their age or illness. People who use health and social care services can be vulnerable because of their care and support needs as they require assistance, care or support and are unable to take care of and protect themselves.

Thinking cap 12.1

Vulnerable people

Think about and make a list of those people who may be deemed a vulnerable adult based on the definition of the term. How long was your list and did it surprise you that the list was so long?

Helping people with their care and providing them with support in order for them to live full lives while being free from abuse and neglect requires a balance between the right to be safe and the right to make informed choices. This includes preventing abuse and minimising risk, but at the same time without taking control away from individuals and also responding appropriately if abuse or neglect has occurred.

Types of harm and abuse

We can all be vulnerable to abuse at some time in our lives. Abuse is about power and control that one individual has over another; it can be a single act or it may continue over months or years. Regardless of whether it is intentional or not it will result in harm to the person. When one person has more power than another, that person can either do things to support the other person to be independent or they may take advantage of their power and this can cause harm to the vulnerable person.

Abuse is a violation of a person's human and civil rights by any other person or persons. It is often (but not always) a crime and can be committed by anyone, anywhere. Often there is more than one type of abuse in any situation, it may not always be intentional and it can be the result of ignorance.

Vulnerable adults may not only experience abuse but also often find it difficult to access services and support to help them live their lives. Table 12.1 highlights the different types of abuse, with a description for each type and the potential signs. You need to know the types of abuse and the indications so that you are able to recognise them, take action and make your concerns known.

Table 12.1 Types of abuse

Type	Description	Indications
Physical	Being hurt or harmed either deliberately or through rough, careless or thoughtless behaviour	Signs of physical abuse could be: • Unexplained bruises • Cuts • Burns • Scalds • Restraint marks • Broken bones • Loss of clumps of hair • Bites
Psychological, emotional abuse or bullying	Being humiliated or put down or made to feel anxious or frightened, being sworn at, being patronised or bullied	A person may become withdrawn, tearful, experience sleep disturbances and have nightmares, experience incontinence, become angry or abusive There may be anxiety, a lack of confidence and low self-esteem. They may start to drink heavily, use drugs, or develop eating disorders
Financial abuse or theft	The misuse of a person's money or possessions (assets)	Signs of financial abuse could be when a person may be unable to pay their bills, buy food and clothing. They may avoid talking about money. Even when they are receiving all their benefits, pension or wages the person may ask to borrow money Valuable possessions may disappear from their home, or they may be pressurised to change a will or make a will
Neglect	Not being given the things needed to feel safe and comfortable	When a person is left dirty, without any clean clothes, or is not fed properly or not given a drink – all may be signs of neglect. They may appear malnourished and dehydrated The person may be denied access to friends and family and social contacts
Sexual abuse	Being made to do something sexual in nature that the vulnerable adult does not want to do or is unable to give consent to	Signs may include the presence of sexually transmitted infection, pregnancy, urinary tract infection, bruising and tears to the thighs, breast area, vagina, penis, anus or mouth and an observation of inappropriate touching. The person's underwear may be bloodstained. There may be pain and discomfort when walking. The person's behaviour may also change
Acts of omission	Failing to provide the care or treatment the person needs	The person's health or medical needs may not be addressed. They may be denied access to aids and adaptations such as hearing aids, walking frames
Discrimination	This is when a person is treated unfairly, e.g. as a result of their ethnicity, gender, sexuality or disability	The person can experience verbal abuse, insults, name calling, hate mail, or other threats Service provision may fail to meet their needs They may be excluded from aspects of service provision
Institutional	Occurs when an organisation or company mistreats people due to poor practices	People may be excluded, mistreated or denied choices by the bad practices They may be denied the opportunity to choose what they want to wear or what they would like to eat or how care is provided. There may be evidence of rigid, inflexible routines

Stop, look, respond 12.2

Other types of abuse

Whilst not always falling within the vulnerable adult criteria, there are other types of abuse. In the table below write notes about these other types of abuse:

Domestic abuse	
Honour-based abuse	
Forced marriage	
Female genital mutilation	

Safeguarding vulnerable adults: the principles

Six principles are associated with the safeguarding of adults, as described in Table 12.2. Applying the six principles of safeguarding where you work can help to ensure that you deliver the best care and support to the people for whom you are responsible. In the organisation where you work there are principles and guidelines available for ensuring that care is safe and effective and people are protected.

Stop, look, respond 12.3

Guidelines, policies and procedures

Familiarise yourself with the guidelines, policies and procedures that are available in your place of work with regards to safeguarding the vulnerable adult and identify the six principles:

1. Empowerment
2. Protection
3. Prevention
4. Proportionality
5. Partnership
6. Accountability

Guidelines should ensure that:

- Services are suitable and fitting to the individual and are non-discriminatory.
- People are permitted to make their own decisions, as far as possible, with support or the provision of advocacy support to help them make choices if appropriate.

Table 12.2   Principles of safeguarding adults

Empowerment	A belief that the person has been involved in person-led decisions and informed consent. The presumption that adults should be in charge of their care and of any decisions that affect their lives
Protection	The support of those in utmost need. Where adults are less able to protect or promote their own interests, reasonable and appropriate measures should be taken to ensure their protection. A dedicated multi-agency approach using multiagency procedures may be required
Prevention	Prevention of harm or abuse is the primary goal working with people to reduce risks of harm or abuse that they find unacceptable. The prevention and avoidance of situations before harm could happen
Proportionality	This includes a balanced and least restrictive option and a response that is appropriate to the risk identified
Partnership	Working within local communities, to prevent, identify and report any signs of neglect or harm to a person
Accountability	The requirement to be accountable for all actions, transparent when providing care and offering support for people and while taking part in safeguarding

- Adults are presumed to have the mental capacity to make informed decisions about their lives, unless an assessment has been undertaken and the person is deemed as not having capacity at that point in time.
- Information is provided, and advice and support are offered, to any identified at-risk adult, in a format that they are able to understand, and that the person's wishes and chosen outcomes are key to any safeguarding decision made about them and their lives.
- Any decision taken by health or social care professionals regarding a person's life should be done in a timely fashion, be reasonable, justified and proportionate to identified risks.

As well as the six principles of safeguarding there should also be a statement that those you care for and support are kept safe and lead lives that are rewarding. The health or support workers should also be provided with information concerning the staff's responsibilities (agreed ways of working). Your organisation should be able to provide evidence that it is taking seriously its responsibilities about safeguarding. There must be information regarding early intervention and ways in which referral to a professional body or safeguarding authority should occur and the circumstances associated with these.

A person-centred approach

Competent adults have a right to make decisions that will have an impact on their lives, even if this could result in the person being exposed to risk. When adults are labelled as 'vulnerable' this can result in stigma, which can lead to assumptions about the person's ability to direct their own lives. This may then lead to paternalism and paternalistic interventions resulting in disempowerment. However, drawing on too narrow a definition of vulnerability could mean losing opportunities to identify those adults who may benefit from additional support.

Understanding the wide range of circumstances in which safeguarding issues can arise can help to address the specific needs of people. This results in a person-centred approach that is based on effective communication and respect for each person's dignity and independence. The person is put at the centre and, with support if needed, is able to choose and control how they want their care and support to be.

Safeguarding Adults Boards

There is a requirement for local authorities to create multi-agency Safeguarding Adults Boards. These boards determine how safeguarding procedures are put into practice in a local area. They encourage information sharing ensuring that care provided meets all the needs of the individual.

The role of the Safeguarding Adults Board is to enhance the quality of life of the vulnerable adults who are at risk of abuse and to progressively improve the services for those in need of protection. The role of the board is to:

- determine safeguarding policy;
- coordinate safeguarding activity between agencies;
- facilitate joint training.

The board consists of relevant agencies that have key statutory roles in the safeguarding of vulnerable adults.

Stop, look, respond 12.4

A multi-agency approach

Good safeguarding requires collaboration and transparency with partner agencies. When a person is in need of protection, a dedicated multi-agency approach using multi-agency procedures may be required. Find out who would make up the multi-agency team and the procedures that they use and are governed by.

Identifying and managing risk

We all take risks every day; sometimes when risks are taken we learn from the consequences. When providing care to others or offering them support, risk taking (risk enablement) becomes part of self-directed care; those providing care can assist people to identify and assess their own risks and realise any potential consequences. Providing support helps the person to take more control over their care, making their own decisions. Being in control, choosing your own risks increases a person's self-confidence.

Thinking cap 12.2

Person-centred care

Person-centred care can help the person to make their own choices, and assess and take risks. It is essential that they understand the consequences of the decisions that they make.

Can you think of any instances/decisions where you have had to help people for whom you care or offer support with regards to understanding the potential consequences of the decisions they had made?

In order to ensure that a person is supported to make a decision the following should be given consideration along with an assessment of the person's abilities:

- Has the person been given all of the important information required to make a decision?
- If there are alternatives available, has the person been made aware of these and been provided with information concerning the alternatives?
- Consider whether if the information was presented differently, the person would be able to understand or process it any better.
- Is the person better able to understand at different times of the day?
- Would the person feel more comfortable in a different place(s) and as such be able to make decisions better?
- Can making the decision wait; can it be delayed until the circumstances are different?
- Would the person be more in control with the assistance of somebody else present to help them to make their decision?

Suspected or disclosed abuse

In all instances priority must be given to ensuring the safety and care of the vulnerable adult. All staff have a duty to report any witnessed or suspected abuse to their line manager. The information should be discussed with social services and every reported case has to be assessed as a matter of urgency in order to decide on an appropriate course of action.

If you suspect abuse or if abuse is disclosed or made known to you then you should know what to do; this is part of the agreed ways of working. Any suspicions of abuse have to be followed up formally and you have a responsibility to respond to any allegations or suspicions by using local workplace safeguarding policies and procedures.

You must be aware of your local multi-agency organisational procedures and the role that is expected of you within these. The procedures will determine the person to whom you should report your concerns and the procedures that will follow.

If a person chooses to disclose abuse to you, then this is because they trust you. If somebody confides in you, regardless what position you hold or your relationship to the person making the disclosure, you have to act. It is not your responsibility to decide if the person is being abused; this is the responsibility of the social work and safeguarding teams. When dealing with suspected abuse this can be distressing and you should consider seeking appropriate support for yourself.

Where disclosure has been made to you, you will need to have an awareness of the feelings that the person may be experiencing and what they may be looking for by disclosing to you. Procedures should be adhered to and must be followed when responding to an adult at risk. Table 12.3 provides a list of issues that should be considered.

If it is an emergency situation you are required to take action to protect the safety and wellbeing of the person being abused. If the person requires any medical help call for a suitably qualified worker; in a community setting you should call 999 to request an ambulance. If you think that any injuries on the person are not accidental then let the worker know this in order for them to preserve any evidence that might be called for in a criminal case. If an offence has been committed the police may need to be contacted and a safeguarding investigation may need to be initiated straightaway.

Ensure that you make a record of what the person has told you; there may be forms available locally to be used enabling you to make the record. The record should be non-biased, and where possible you should use the person's own words; by doing this you will not forget any details.

Table 12.3   Issues that should be considered when a person discloses

- Let the person know that you are taking them seriously
- Listen carefully to what is being told to you, stay calm, attempt to obtain as clear a picture as you can. However, avoid asking too many questions at this stage
- Never give promises of being completely confidential
- Make it clear that you have a duty to inform your manager or other designated person, and that there is a possibility that concerns could be shared with others who have a part to play in protecting the person
- Explain to the person that they will be involved in decisions about what will happen
- Reassure the person that you will try to take steps to protect them from any further abuse or neglect
- If the person has any specific communication needs, provide support and information in a way that they can understand
- Never be judgmental or jump to conclusions

A factual report is required, not one that contains your views. Follow local policy regarding report writing. There will be a requirement for you to sign and date it.

Reporting concerns

The Public Interest Disclosure Act 1998 (PIDA) protects the health of social care workers by providing a solution if they suffer a workplace punishment for raising a concern that they believe to be genuine. The Care Act 2014 places a duty on local authorities to make enquiries if a person is being abused or neglected, or is at risk of abuse or neglect in their area. You have to report things that you feel are not right, or are illegal, including any of the following:

- when there is a risk to someone's health and safety;
- if the environment is unsafe;
- a criminal offence has been or is likely to be committed;
- the organisation you work for is not obeying the law or they are covering up wrongdoings.

You might have serious concerns about what is happening at your workplace, and the issues you are concerned about might have a negative impact on people receiving care or support or those you work with. But it can be difficult to know what to do in these circumstances. Raising the matter might make you feel as if you are being unfaithful to co-workers, to your manager or to your organisation. But you have to behave in a professional manner and put the people for whom you care or offer support to first; keeping them safe is your priority.

If you have concerns, in the first instance you should try to resolve these within your organisation. You will be able to justify raising a genuine concern about the safety of people or standards of care if you do so honestly and reasonably, even if you are mistaken. If you feel you are unable to do this or you believe that nobody is listening to you, then speak to someone who is independent or external to your organisation, for example your trade union.

If a health or social care worker is concerned that vulnerable adults using a service are not being cared for in a way that keeps them safe, they can raise their concern with the local authority (local council); they can also inform a regulatory body such as the Care Quality Commission or report it to the police.

It is essential that you are familiar with your organisation's policies and procedures so that you know what to do if you see abuse or if abuse is disclosed to you.

Table 12.4 outlines the immediate action to be taken if there is no policy or procedure in place or available. The steps described in Table 12.4 should be used as a framework for response in an emergency.

Stop, look, respond 12.5

Policies and procedures

You have to know what your role and responsibilities are in relation to safeguarding adults. This information should be provided to you and it may be in the form of policies and procedures. In your own organisation where could you find information and advice regarding your role and responsibilities in preventing and protecting individuals from harm and abuse? Make a list that identifies the type(s) of information that is available you. Also identify who you would go to for advice regarding the safeguarding of adults.

Table 12.4   Immediate action to be taken if you see abuse or if abuse is disclosed to you

- Make an immediate evaluation of the risk, take steps to ensure that the adult is not in immediate danger
- If there is a need for emergency medical treatment, dial 999 (or the emergency response number in your location) for an ambulance. If you suspect that the injury is non-accidental, inform the paramedics, so that appropriate measures are taken to preserve any potential forensic evidence. If possible, establish with the adult at risk the action that they wish you to take
- Contact the police if a crime has been or may have been committed. Alert your manager
- Do not disturb or move articles that could be used in evidence and secure the area, e.g. by locking a room
- As far as is possible, make sure that others are not at risk

Chapter summary

- A vulnerable adult is described as a person who is in need of assistance, care or support and is unable to take care of and protect themselves.
- Abuse can take place anytime and anywhere.
- Adult safeguarding protects those adults with care and support needs from abuse, harm or neglect.
- Safeguarding balances the right to be safe along with the right to make informed choices.
- We all have a role to play in safeguarding.
- You should always ensure that your actions or omissions do not harm a person's health or wellbeing.
- There are seven types of abuse and you should be able to identify and know the signs that abuse may be occurring.
- Policies and procedures are available in the place where you work providing guidance on prevention and recognising the signs and symptoms of abuse as well as procedures to be followed if and when abuse has happened.
- Safeguarding Adults Boards set out the ways in which safeguarding procedures are put into practice in your local area.
- Risk enablement is a part of self-directed care and support and involves supporting individuals to identify and assess their own risks, enabling the person to take the risks they choose.
- Any suspicions of abuse must be followed up in a formal way.
- You have a responsibility to respond to allegations or suspicions in association with your workplace safeguarding policies and procedures.
- In an emergency you must take action to protect the safety and wellbeing of the person who has been abused or alleges abuse.
- If the person requires medical assistance call for a suitably qualified worker or dial 999 for an ambulance.

Case scenario 12.1

Mr Darcy

Mr Darcy was recovering from a stroke and being cared for in a nursing home. He was making a slow recovery and he was quite confused. Gradually he regained the ability to walk but was prone to wandering beyond the confines of the main building. Outside the home was a busy road and those caring for Mr Darcy were worried about his wellbeing. Staff were also concerned about restricting his freedom of movement and at the same time worried that he might come to some harm. In discussing his care with Mr Darcy, the care team decided that although Mr Darcy was confused at times, he seemed to understand what he was doing. They spoke with him about the potential risks that he was exposing himself to.

Mr Darcy used to be a construction worker when he was active and worked outdoors. Hence at times he felt restricted and uncomfortable in his room. Mr Darcy was able to understand the risks involved and that his freedom to get out and walk and to get fresh air was important to him. After several discussions with Mr Darcy and those who cared for him it was determined that he retained capacity and he was aware of the risks. It would have been wrong, as well as unlawful, to introduce restrictions beyond the ordinary security measures needed to keep all the residents safe.

A written record of the discussions and of the risk assessment of Mr Darcy's capacity to manage the risks was made.

Resource file

Care Inspectorate
One of the Care Inspectorate's regulatory and scrutiny functions is to ensure that vulnerable people are safe (Scotland).
http://www.gov.scot/Topics/Health/Support-Social-Care/Care-Inspectorate

Care and Social Services Inspectorate Wales
Responsible for inspecting social care and social services to make sure that they are safe for the people who use them (Wales).
http://cssiw.org.uk/raiseaconcern/?lang=en

Regulation and Quality Improvement Authority
Independent body responsible for monitoring and inspecting the availability and quality of health and social care services (Northern Ireland).
https://www.rqia.org.uk/what-we-do/inspect/mental-health-learning-disability-services/

Care Quality Commission
Monitors, inspects and regulates services ensuring they meet fundamental standards of quality and safety (England).
http://www.cqc.org.uk

Chapter 13

Safeguarding children

Care certificate outcomes

1. To safeguard children.

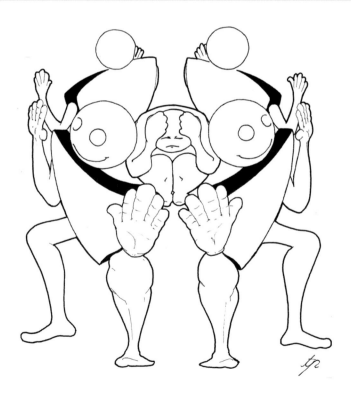

Fundamentals of Care: A Textbook for Health and Social Care Assistants, First Edition. Ian Peate.
© 2017 John Wiley & Sons Ltd. Published 2017 by John Wiley & Sons Ltd.

Take stock

Rate your current knowledge and skills prior to reading this chapter. Put a tick in the box that you think applies to you with regards to the standard being discussed:

Key:

I know this
I have a good level of knowledge or skills regarding this aspect of the standard. I make use of the knowledge and skills identified on a regular basis, feeling confident in my ability and performance. I do not need a refresher.

Satisfactory
My level of knowledge and standard of skills meet the criteria associated with the standard. I use the skills and knowledge from time to time. I might not always feel confident in my capability. I would benefit from a refresher.

I require a review
I do not feel that I have the skills and/or the knowledge that would enable me to meet the standard in a confident and competent way. The knowledge and skills I used to have are no longer valid. I will require a refresher.

This is new to me
I have never worked in a caring role before or I have never covered this topic before. I will need further training and development in this area.

Standard	Self-assessment			
Recognise potential indicators of child maltreatment	☐ I know this	☐ Satisfactory	☐ I should review this	☐ This is new to me
Understand the impact a parent's/carer's physical and mental health can have on the wellbeing of a child or young person, including domestic violence	☐ I know this	☐ Satisfactory	☐ I should review this	☐ This is new to me
Understand the importance of children's rights concerning safeguarding/child protection	☐ I know this	☐ Satisfactory	☐ I should review this	☐ This is new to me
Describe the action to be taken if you have concerns	☐ I know this	☐ Satisfactory	☐ I should review this	☐ This is new to me
Demonstrate an understanding of the risks associated with the internet and online social networking	☐ I know this	☐ Satisfactory	☐ I should review this	☐ This is new to me
Understand the basic knowledge of legislation and safeguarding children	☐ I know this	☐ Satisfactory	☐ I should review this	☐ This is new to me

Introduction

All those who work with children ('child/children' in this chapter refers to any person up to the age of 18 years), including health and social care support workers, have a responsibility to keep children safe and to protect them from harm.

Thinking cap 13.1

Working with children

Can you think of any other groups who work with children who also have a duty to keep them safe and to protect them from harm?

Safeguarding children, as with adults, is everyone's responsibility. Children should be protected from abuse and from any injury that could impact on their health, wellbeing and development. Some children are in particular need of safeguarding, for example those who are disabled, those who have educational or other specific additional needs, and those who suffer signs of child abuse, substance abuse or domestic violence. The Children Acts 1989 and 2004 charge local authorities with the responsibility of providing services for children who are in need for the intentions of safeguarding and promoting their welfare. Children should be protected from maltreatment (abuse) and any impairment that could interfere with their health and development. Furthermore, we all have to ensure that children grow up with safe and effective care and support.

Care and support workers are well placed to identify those children and young people who may be at risk and to act in order to safeguard them. You should be familiar with local referral arrangements.

Thinking cap 13.2

Making referrals

Do you know what your local referral arrangements are?

Whilst written procedures, protocols and guidance are available to help support the health and social care worker these will not in themselves protect children. What is required is a skilled, competent, confident and committed workforce that is willing to act against abuse and neglect in an organised way as well as embracing multidisciplinary and multi-agency ways of working.

Each child is an individual in a relationship with his or her parents, wider family, school, friends, neighbourhood, society and culture. Traumatic events such as abuse or maltreatment can have a negative impact upon a child's development. Children have the ability to recover from abuse or other negative experiences and the support they receive is crucial to this, as well as the seriousness of the harm they suffered and its duration. Early identification of risk and intervention tells us that children can recover from abuse and go on to reach their full potential.

Safeguarding and welfare

Safeguarding and promoting welfare are defined as:

- protecting children from maltreatment;
- preventing damage to a child's health or development;

- ensuring that children grow up in conditions that are consistent with the provision of safe and effective care;
- taking action to help all children have the best life chances, good health and social care.

Safeguarding is a preventative act that promotes the welfare of children by offering them protection from harm and understanding the potential risks to their safety and security. Child protection is the act of protecting those children who are suffering or may be suffering from substantial harm due to acts of abuse or neglect.

 ## Stop, look, respond 13.1

Safeguarding

Safeguarding covers a wide range of levels. In the table below write notes on the three specific areas of safeguarding.

Area of safeguarding	Description
Universal safeguarding	
Targeted safeguarding	
Specialist safeguarding	

Child abuse and maltreatment

Child abuse is any offence that causes or could cause considerable emotional or physical harm to a child. The signs, symptoms and behaviours or indicators discussed here do not necessarily mean that a child is being abused but they may mean that you have a reason to be concerned.

Regardless of the type of abuse, all forms of abuse will lead to a change in behaviour of the child who is being abused. Behaviour changes may mean that a child becomes:

- withdrawn;
- shy;
- easily scared;
- overactive/overexcited/boisterous;
- aggressive/violent;
- attention-seeking or keen to please.

Other pointers can include:

- depression;
- anxiety;
- self-harm/self-injury;
- eating disorder;
- going back or regressing to younger behavioural patterns.

Further concerns may include:

- the child failing to attend school regularly;
- the child being admitted to several different accident and emergency departments or GP drop-in centres/walk-in centres.

It is important to note that not all children will display the same symptoms, and often there is more than one type of abuse occurring (coexisting), such as physical and emotional abuse.

Impact of parents or carers on a child's health and wellbeing

There are a number of factors regarding parents or carers that may increase the risk of a child being abused. Risk factors can include:

- domestic violence;
- drug and alcohol misuse;
- mental health problems;
- deprivation;
- single-parent family;
- young age of parent.

The main categories of abuse are:

- physical;
- sexual;
- emotional;
- neglect;
- fabricated or induced illness.

Fabricated or induced illness (FII)

This describes behaviours by a parent or carer that can result in harm to the child, including deliberately inducing symptoms by administering medication or other substances, or by intentional suffocation. Meddling with treatments may take the form of overdosing, withholding the child's medication, or interfering with equipment being used in the care of the child. There may also be claims that the child has symptoms that cannot be verified, or exaggeration of symptoms that could result in the child having to undergo unnecessary investigations or treatments. Falsification of test results and observation charts, obtaining specialist treatments or equipment that are not required, and making allegations of psychological illness can also feature in FII relating to a child. FII can cause significant, long-term or permanent injury as well as long-term impairment of a child's psychological and emotional development, and may even result in the death of a child.

Types of abuse

A child may be maltreated, abused or neglected by somebody if they are inflicting harm on them, or if they fail to act to prevent harm. The abuse of a child can take place in a family or in an institutional or community setting, by those who are known to the child or by others, for example, via the internet. An adult or adults, or another child or children, may abuse the child.

Thinking cap 13.3

Preventing harm

Reflect now on how failing to prevent harm to a child can be seen as a form of abuse.

Physical abuse

This is a form of abuse that can involve hitting, shaking, throwing, poisoning, burning or scald-ing, drowning, suffocating or otherwise causing physical harm to a child. Physical harm could also be caused when a parent or carer makes up the symptoms of an illness, or deliberately causes illness in a child; this is also known as fabricated or induced illness (see earlier).

Emotional abuse

Emotional abuse is defined as the ongoing emotional maltreatment or emotional neglect of a child that will lead to severe and persistent harmful effects on the child's emotional develop-ment. This can involve telling a child that they are meaningless or unloved or inadequate or that they are only valued insofar as they meet the needs of another person. It can involve not giving the child their chances to voice their views or opinions, purposely silencing them, or ridiculing what they say or how they communicate. Expectations may be imposed on the child that are inappropriate for the stage of her/his development, including interactions that are beyond a child's developmental capability, as well as overprotection and limitation of exploration and learning, or blocking the child from taking part in normal social interaction. Abuse may also involve witnessing the ill-treatment of another person. Serious bullying (including cyberbully-ing) can result in the child regularly feeling frightened or in danger, or involve exploitation (taking advantage of a child's vulnerability to treat them badly for the abuser's benefit) or corruption of the child. All types of maltreatment of a child involve some level of emotional abuse, but such abuse can happen alone.

Sexual abuse

Sexual abuse involves forcing or enticing a child to engage in sexual activities. This may not necessarily involve a high level of violence, whether or not the child is aware of what is happen-ing. The activities can concern physical contact, including assault by penetration (rape or oral sex) or non-penetrative activity, for example, masturbation, kissing, rubbing and touching outside of clothing. They may also include non-contact activities, for example involving a child in looking at, or in the production of, sexual images, watching sexual activities, encouraging a child to act or perform in sexually inappropriate ways, or grooming a child in preparation for abuse (including via the internet). It is not only adult males who carry out sexual abuse; women can also commit acts of sexual abuse, as well as other children.

Neglect

This form of abuse involves the persistent failure to meet a child's basic physical and/or psycho-logical needs and results in serious harm to the child's health or development. Neglect can also occur during pregnancy, for example as a result of the mother's substance abuse, and substance

Stop, look, respond 13.2

PANTS

The NSPCC has introduced the underwear rule. This is a very easy way for parents to explain the Underwear Rule to their child:

Privates are private
Always remember your body belongs to you
No means no
Talk about secrets that upset you
Speak up, someone can help

Using the underwear rule a child can learn that those parts of their body that are covered by underwear are private. It should be explained to the child that no one should ask to see or touch their private parts or ask them to look at or touch anyone else's. However, there are times when doctors, nurses or family members might have to. Explain that this is OK, but that those people should always explain why, and first ask the child if it is OK.

misuse can have a serious impact on children in the family. When a child is born, neglect may involve a parent or carer failing to:

- provide adequate food, clothing and shelter;
- protect a child from physical and emotional harm or danger;
- ensure adequate supervision;
- ensure access to appropriate medical care or treatment.

It could also include neglect of, or unresponsiveness to, a child's basic emotional needs.

Radicalisation

This refers to the process by which a child comes to support terrorism and hold extremist beliefs related to terrorist groups. The child is taught extreme, often violent ideas based on political, social or religious beliefs. A child may be exposed to messages about terrorism through a family member or friend, a religious school or group, or through social media and the internet. This creates the risk of a child being drawn into criminal activity as well as exposure to significant harm.

Trafficking

This means having control over recruiting, moving or receiving a child through force or threat, abduction, coercion, deception or intimidation to take advantage of them. Exploitation can include prostitution, sexual exploitation, forced labour or services, slavery or practices similar to slavery.

Female genital mutilation (FGM)

This is a highly complex form of abuse. Female genital mutilation comprises all procedures involving partial or total removal of the external female genitalia or other injury to the female genital organs for non-medical reasons. It has no health benefits and harms girls in many ways.

Normal female genital tissue is removed and damaged; this interferes with the natural function of a girl's body, and is a form of abuse.

The age at which girls undergo female genital mutilation varies according to the community in which they live. The procedure may be carried out when the girl is newborn, during childhood or adolescence, just before marriage or during the first pregnancy. In the majority of cases, however, it takes place between the ages of 5 and 8 years.

Stop, look, respond 13.3

Female genital mutilation (FGM)

FGM is illegal; it is a form of child abuse and violates the rights of the child. It is not approved by any religion. There are four types of FGM; describe them in the table below.

Type of FGM	Description
Female genital mutilation type 1	
Female genital mutilation type 2	
Female genital mutilation type 3	
Female genital mutilation type 4	

Gang abuse

Sexual, physical and emotional abuse of children by gangs and groups can occur; the use of weapons is often associated with gangs. Some children's experiences of familial abuse can increase their vulnerability to exploitation. Mobile phones, social networking sites and other forms of technology are used as channels through which gangs groom, bully and pursue victims. Violence is used to keep victims controlled, as well as oral and anal rape as a form of humiliation and subjugation.

Children living in residential care are known to be especially vulnerable, particularly if placements have broken down or the child has a record of running away. But children from stable homes who appear to be doing well at school can also be drawn unconsciously into exploitation and/or gang activity.

Children and social media

The internet has brought with it a number of advantages for entertainment, communication and education. There are also potential risks to a child's safety and security, creating opportunities for the child to be exposed to situations for which they are emotionally and psychologically unprepared. Examples include images of abuse, pornography or violence including child abuse and sexual violence, as well as communication with people or groups who may be intent on harm.

The internet may be used to befriend and groom children as an opening to sexual exploitation. 'Sexting' is the exchange of self-produced sexually explicit images through mobile picture messages or webcams via the internet. Posting or publishing these images could also potentially expose the child to exploitation, bullying, humiliation and further harm.

Stop, look, respond 13.4

Signs and symptoms of abuse

In the table below consider the various types of abuse and the symptoms that may accompany them – remember to take into account the child's physical and psychological wellbeing.

Type of abuse	Signs, symptoms and pointers
Physical	
Emotional	
Sexual	
Neglect	
Radicalisation	
Trafficking	
Female genital mutilation	
Gang abuse	

Stop, look, respond 13.5

Staying safe on social media

Children and young people may present to a service such as general practice with low mood, sleep disturbance, behavioural disorders, self-harm or suicidal thoughts or intent as a reaction to cyberbullying.

Cyberbullying can lead to depression, isolation, self-harm and in severe cases suicide. How might you help a child stay safe whilst using social media?

The rights of the child

The United Nations Convention on the Rights of the Child makes clear that children have the right to be protected from being hurt and mistreated, physically or mentally. Governments have a duty to ensure that children are properly cared for and are protected from violence, abuse and neglect by their parents or anyone else who cares for them.

Stop, look, respond 13.6

United Nations Convention on the Rights of the Child

Access the United Nations Convention on the Rights of the Child (UK UNICEF): http://www.unicef.org.uk

Consider the various articles of the convention and draw out what a child-centred perspective means.

It is important that you understand the rights of the child. Although you may not directly care for or support children, through your work you may come into contact with them. You must remember that you have a duty to promote and uphold the privacy, dignity, rights, health and wellbeing of those who use health and social care services as well as their carers; children may also be carers.

With regards to the welfare of children there are a number of pieces of legislation (laws) that should be taken into account as well as your own organisation's policies and procedures and agreed ways of working. Table 13.1 provides an overview of some laws in England that may impact on the welfare of children.

The Children Act 1989 introduced the rule that the welfare of the child is supreme. The 1989 Act defined parental responsibility as having 'all the rights, duties, powers, responsibilities, and authority'. The Children Act 2004 ensures that the welfare of the child is the healthcare provider's first concern; this takes precedence over maintaining confidentiality when these are in conflict. Health and social care workers are well placed to identify children who may be at risk. The principles of safeguarding across the four UK countries are similar, and child protection frameworks for the UK countries have detailed definitions of safeguarding, child protection and types of abuse.

In the UK the Human Rights Act 1998 provides various fundamental rights to every person. They include:

- the right to life;
- freedom from torture or degrading treatment;
- the right to education;
- the right to liberty and security;
- protection from discrimination.

What to do if you have concerns of suspected or alleged abuse

Providing early help is more effective in promoting a child's welfare than reacting later. Early help means providing support as soon as a problem emerges, at any point in a child's life, from the foundation years through to the teenage years. Early help can prevent further problems arising. If you have any concerns and are worried about a child:

Table 13.1   An overview of some elements of relevant legislation that may impact on the welfare of children

Legislation	Description
The Children Act 1989	Protects the welfare of children who are at risk as well as those children who might be in need of services. Details the actions required if there is any suspicion that a child is at risk of harm or in need of support
The Children Act 2004	Describes the services that a child may access. A duty is placed on local authorities and their partners to cooperate and ensure, where possible, that services work together in producing a joint plan that has been developed in partnership with the parents and children. This is the Common Assessment Framework. Local Safeguarding Children Boards and joint databases are encouraged under the auspices of this act
The Sexual Offences Act 2003	There are two parts; the first part states what is considered a sexual offence, including physical and non-physical contact. The Act also defines sexual offences against those children under 13 years and under 16 years of age. The age of consent is set at 16, unless you hold a position of trust in relation to the young person, e.g. as their worker, teacher or trainer, and if this is the case the age of consent is 18 years. Part two of the act addresses the sex offenders register and also civil protective orders
The Care Act 2014	This brings together in a single Act care and support legislation with a new emphasis on wellbeing principles at its heart. Whilst the Care Act focuses on adults who are in need of support and their carers, there are also some provisions for children and young carers. Children who care for their parents in their own home are made part of their parent's needs assessment, which establishes the support and help they need
The Children and Families Act 2014	Aims to provide young carers with the same help and support as adult carers receive. Carers under the age of 18 years have the right to have their support needs assessed and local authorities will help them in caring for a family member
Safeguarding Vulnerable Groups Act 2006	Established a single body to make decisions about those who should be barred from working with children and to maintain a list of these individuals
Female Genital Mutilation Act 2003	In 2015 the Serious Crimes Act together with this Act makes provisions for FGM Protection Orders and the legal duty for regulated social care and health professionals and teachers to make a report to the police if a girl under 18 tells them she has undergone an act of FGM, or if they observe physical signs that a girl under 18 has undergone FGM

- Immediately report your concerns to your manager.
- Record your concerns (document them) but ensure this is factual; sign, write your name and date it.
- If you think that the process is taking too long then call the police by dialing 999. Action can then be taken quickly to have the child removed to somewhere safe.
- Ensure that you adhere to the safeguarding policies and procedures that are used in your organisation. These set out clearly how you should act if abuse is suspected or alleged.

An allegation of abuse might be made by a child, stating that they have been abused by someone or a family member, friend, worker or someone else. The allegation could be about abuse happening now or in the past. Any allegations made have to be reported and investigated. Local policies and procedures should provide information about:

- signs and symptoms of abuse;
- how to make an appropriate response to the victim;
- how the report has to be managed (lines of reporting);
- important telephone numbers you can use in order to feel confident when dealing with issues.

You must not hesitate if you have any concerns about a child being abused. Your role is not to judge situations, people or issues; this is the duty of others such as the police and social workers. However, if you fail to alert them, they are unable to act.

Stop, look, respond 13.7

Local policy and procedure

Locate your own organisation's policies and procedures that are related to the protection of children. Take note of how you should proceed if you suspect abuse or if there are any allegations being made concerning the safety of a child.

How would you be required to make a report regarding your concerns; are there any templates available?

In your workplace who is the person responsible for child protection?

Make a note of key contacts and telephone numbers you might need if you have any worries or concerns.

Escalating concerns

If the concerns you have raised have not been taken seriously and no action has been taken, report your concerns either to a senior manager or to the person who is responsible for child protection in your workplace. Child protection records should always be shared with the parents/carers unless it is they who are the cause for concern. You can seek advice and support from other workers, your manager, the child's parent/carer, the NSPCC or Children's Services. Appropriate action will be taken by your manager in accordance with your organisation's agreed ways of working, and usually this will entail contacting the relevant agencies such as the police, the health visitor or the education department.

Chapter summary

- The care or support worker should be able to recognise potential indicators of child maltreatment – physical, emotional, or sexual abuse and neglect including radicalisation, child trafficking and female genital mutilation.
- Understanding the impact a parent's/carer's physical and mental health can have on the wellbeing of a child or young person, including the impact of domestic violence, is essential in assisting children in need.
- Understanding children's rights in the safeguarding/child protection context helps in ensuring children are protected.
- Agreed ways of working, and local and national policies dictate what action needs to be taken if you have concerns, including who you should report your concerns to and who to seek advice from should you need to.
- Providing early help is more effective in promoting a child's welfare as opposed to reacting later.
- If you have any concerns and are worried about a child, immediately report your concerns to your manager, and record your concerns.

- If you think that the process is taking too long then call the police so that action can be taken quickly to have the child removed to a place of safety.
- Ensure that you adhere to the safeguarding policies and procedures that are used in your organisation.
- The internet and online social networking have made great strides with regards to communication, education and entertainment, but also come with associated risks.
- There are several elements of law in place to offer support and care in order to ensure that a child's physical and psychological wellbeing is enhanced.

Case scenario 13.1

Karly

Karly is 15 years old; she is binge drinking and stays out late at night with her friends. Karly's mum is worried about her. Karly's relationship with her mother has deteriorated and Karly is occasionally violent and aggressive towards her younger brothers and sisters. She has a new boyfriend who is aged 19 years; he buys Karly gifts, which recently included a brand new state-of-the-art smart phone. Karly has recently attended for sexual health advice and has been diagnosed with chlamydia – a sexually transmitted infection.

What, if any, further steps need to be taken with regards to safeguarding Karly?
    Why might childhood sexual exploitation be considered in this scenario?

Resource file

The Child Exploitation and Online Protection Centre (CEOP)
CEOP works with child protection partners throughout the UK and internationally to identify the main threats to children, and coordinates activity against these threats to bring offenders to account.
https://ceop.police.uk

National Society for the Protection of Cruelty to Children (NSPCC)
The NSPCC stands up for children by finding the best ways to prevent abuse and neglect and influencing government to take action.
https://www.nspcc.org.uk

NSPCC Child Line
0800 1111

United Nations Convention on the Rights of the Child
UNICEF promotes the rights and wellbeing of every child, in all it does. It works in 190 countries and territories, translating that commitment into practical action, focusing special effort on reaching the most vulnerable and excluded children, to the benefit of all children, everywhere.
http://www.unicef.org.uk/UNICEFs-Work/UN-Convention/

Chapter 14

Basic life support

Care certificate outcomes

1. Provide basic life support.

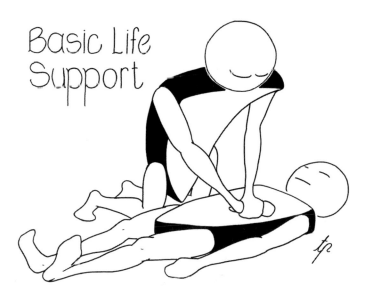

Fundamentals of Care: A Textbook for Health and Social Care Assistants, First Edition. Ian Peate.
© 2017 John Wiley & Sons Ltd. Published 2017 by John Wiley & Sons Ltd.

Take stock

Rate your current knowledge and skills prior to reading this chapter. Put a tick in the box that you think applies to you with regards to the standard being discussed:

Key:
I know this   I have a good level of knowledge or skills regarding this aspect of the standard. I make use of the knowledge and skills identified on a regular basis, feeling confident in my ability and performance. I do not need a refresher.
Satisfactory   My level of knowledge and standard of skills meet the criteria associated with the standard. I use the skills and knowledge from time to time. I might not always feel confident in my capability. I would benefit from a refresher.
I require a review   I do not feel that I have the skills and/or the knowledge that would enable me to meet the standard in a confident and competent way. The knowledge and skills I used to have are no longer valid. I will require a refresher.
This is new to me   I have never worked in a caring role before or I have never covered this topic before. I will need further training and development in this area.

Standard	Self-assessment			
Understand the importance of checking for risks to the person, any bystanders and myself	☐ I know this	☐ Satisfactory	☐ I should review this	☐ This is new to me
Describe how to assess that the person is unresponsive	☐ I know this	☐ Satisfactory	☐ I should review this	☐ This is new to me
Explain how to open the person's airway	☐ I know this	☐ Satisfactory	☐ I should review this	☐ This is new to me
Describe how to establish the absence of normal breathing	☐ I know this	☐ Satisfactory	☐ I should review this	☐ This is new to me
Discuss the ways in which to alert the ambulance service	☐ I know this	☐ Satisfactory	☐ I should review this	☐ This is new to me
Describe how to perform chest compressions	☐ I know this	☐ Satisfactory	☐ I should review this	☐ This is new to me
Describe how to give rescue breaths	☐ I know this	☐ Satisfactory	☐ I should review this	☐ This is new to me
Discuss the way to maintain CPR with the correct ratio of chest compressions to rescue breaths	☐ I know this	☐ Satisfactory	☐ I should review this	☐ This is new to me

Introduction

When a person has a cardiac arrest, basic life support (BLS) can be provided to help their chance of survival. Providing chest compressions will pump blood from the heart around the body, ensuring the tissues and brain continue to receive a good oxygen supply. Basic life support is one of the most important skills you will develop as a health or social care worker.

Basic life support refers to the maintenance of a clear airway and support of breathing and circulation in cases of cardiac arrest. This is performed without the use of equipment (you may have a simple airway device or protective shield available). Cardiopulmonary resuscitation (CPR) is the combination of chest compression and rescue breathing and forms the basis of BLS.

The chances of survival after cardiac arrest are increased when the event is witnessed and when a bystander institutes CPR before the arrival of the emergency services. The best chance of a successful outcome is if chest compressions are started as soon as cardiac arrest is diagnosed. Chest compressions should be given with minimal interruptions at the recommended rate and depth, and accompanied by artificial ventilation in accordance with the current guidelines. The community response to cardiac arrest is critical to saving lives. Strengthening this response to cardiac arrest by training and empowering more bystanders to perform CPR and by increasing the use of automated external defibrillators can at least double the chances of survival and could save thousands of lives each year.

The heart

The heart has four chambers and is responsible for pumping the blood around the body under pressure. As heart muscle (myocardium) contracts it ejects the blood from the aorta (the largest blood vessel in the body) to the rest of the body. Figure 14.1 provides an illustration of the heart and blood flow.

The lungs

Both lungs take in air that is inhaled from the atmosphere. The lungs make up part of the respiratory system, which supplies oxygen to all parts of the body. When we take a breath in (inhale) we breathe in a mixture of:

- nitrogen (79%);
- oxygen (20%);
- other gases (1%).

When we breathe out we exhale a mixture of:

- carbon dioxide (4%);
- nitrogen (79%);
- oxygen (16%);
- other gases (1%).

Figure 14.2 provides an overview of the respiratory system.

Basic life support

This chapter provides the reader with an understanding of BLS; for some this will be a refresher concerning their knowledge of BLS. It is important that those who may be present at the scene of a cardiac arrest, particularly lay bystanders, should have learnt the correct resuscitation skills and be able to put them into practice. The organisation where you work should provide you with training, and this may be a part of mandatory training.

A step-by-step approach should be undertaken when delivering BLS; you should deliver the appropriate steps in the correct order. The outcome for the person depends on providing effective high-quality BLS as well as prompt access to a defibrillator. The Resuscitation Council United Kingdom provides a step-by-step guide for adult BLS reflecting up-to-date guidance.

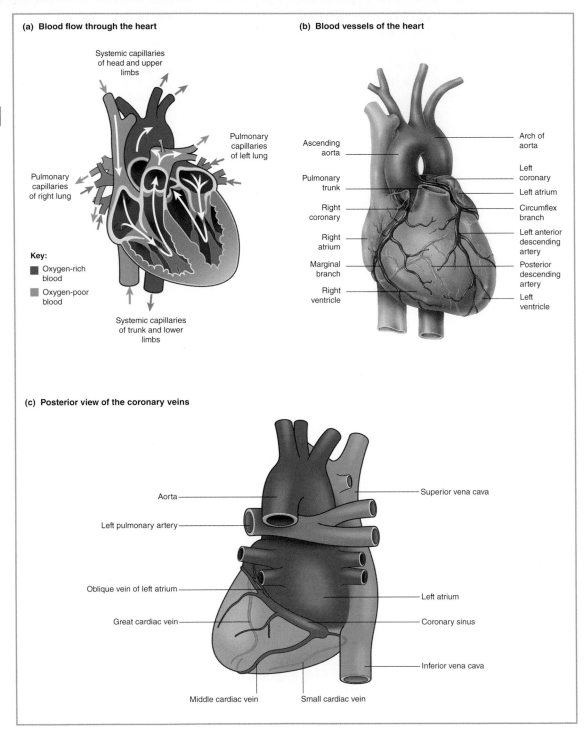

(a) **Blood flow through the heart**

Systemic capillaries of head and upper limbs

Pulmonary capillaries of left lung

Pulmonary capillaries of right lung

Key:
- Oxygen-rich blood
- Oxygen-poor blood

Systemic capillaries of trunk and lower limbs

(b) **Blood vessels of the heart**

Ascending aorta

Pulmonary trunk

Right coronary

Right atrium

Marginal branch

Right ventricle

Arch of aorta

Left coronary

Left atrium

Circumflex branch

Left anterior descending artery

Posterior descending artery

Left ventricle

(c) **Posterior view of the coronary veins**

Aorta

Left pulmonary artery

Oblique vein of left atrium

Great cardiac vein

Superior vena cava

Left atrium

Coronary sinus

Inferior vena cava

Middle cardiac vein

Small cardiac vein

Figure 14.1 The heart and blood flow. *Source*: Peate, I., Wild, K. & Nair, M. (eds) (2014) *Nursing Practice: Knowledge and Care*. Reproduced with permission of John Wiley & Sons, Ltd.

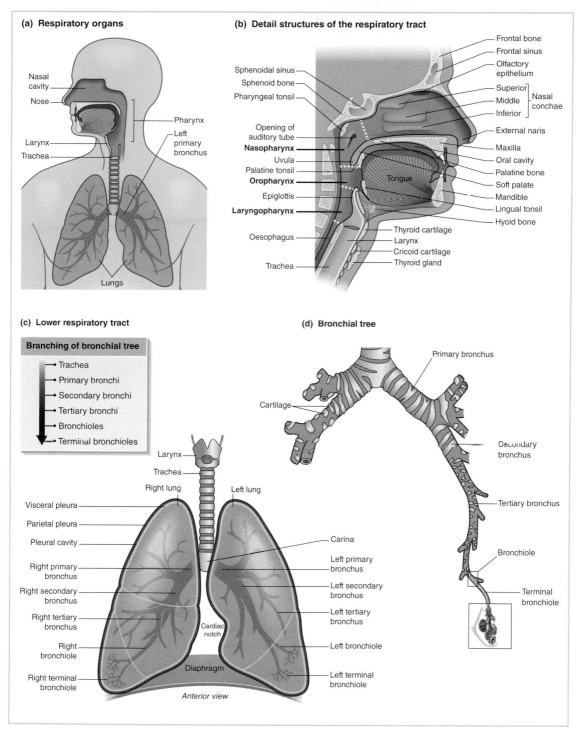

(a) Respiratory organs

Nasal cavity
Nose
Pharynx
Larynx
Trachea
Left primary bronchus
Lungs

(b) Detail structures of the respiratory tract

Sphenoidal sinus
Sphenoid bone
Pharyngeal tonsil
Opening of auditory tube
Nasopharynx
Uvula
Palatine tonsil
Oropharynx
Epiglottis
Laryngopharynx
Oesophagus
Trachea

Frontal bone
Frontal sinus
Olfactory epithelium
Superior
Middle
Inferior
Nasal conchae
External naris
Maxilla
Oral cavity
Palatine bone
Soft palate
Mandible
Lingual tonsil
Hyoid bone
Tongue
Thyroid cartilage
Larynx
Cricoid cartilage
Thyroid gland

(c) Lower respiratory tract

Branching of bronchial tree
- Trachea
- Primary bronchi
- Secondary bronchi
- Tertiary bronchi
- Bronchioles
- Terminal bronchioles

Larynx
Trachea
Right lung
Left lung
Visceral pleura
Parietal pleura
Pleural cavity
Right primary bronchus
Right secondary bronchus
Right tertiary bronchus
Right bronchiole
Right terminal bronchiole
Cardiac notch
Diaphragm
Carina
Left primary bronchus
Left secondary bronchus
Left tertiary bronchus
Left bronchiole
Left terminal bronchiole
Anterior view

(d) Bronchial tree

Cartilage
Primary bronchus
Secondary bronchus
Tertiary bronchus
Bronchiole
Terminal bronchiole

Figure 14.2 An overview of the respiratory system. *Source for (a), (b) and (c)*: Peate, I., Wild, K. & Nair, M. (eds) (2014) *Nursing Practice: Knowledge and Care*. Reproduced with permission of John Wiley & Sons, Ltd. *Source for (d)*: Peate, I. and Nair, M. (2011) *Fundamentals of Anatomy and Physiology for Student Nurses*. Reproduced with permission of John Wiley & Sons, Ltd.

It is important for health and social care providers to understand how to perform BLS. Retention of BLS knowledge declines over time and this has the potential to reduce competence. There is a need for regular updates of BLS to maintain current knowledge and skills.

Thinking cap 14.1

Undertake BLS training

Have you undertaken BLS training? When was the last time you undertook BLS training? When are you due for a BLS refresher?

In performing BLS the following requirements apply:

- Undertake a rapid assessment of the person whom you suspect has experienced cardiac arrest; this is then followed by BLS.
- BLS must be carried out without delay as this can ensure best outcomes.
- BLS is a structured approach that supports breathing and circulation.
- The health and social care worker must maintain the correct techniques for BLS; these will include basic airway management, compressions of the chest and ventilations.

When a person is unconscious it needs to be established quickly if the person is breathing normally or not breathing. Opening and maintaining the airway can achieve this. When approaching a person you must undertake a primary survey; this is an initial assessment. The primary survey must be carried out using a systematic process of approach, which requires you to identify and deal with immediate and/or life-threatening conditions. The acronym DRSABCD can be used (Table 14.1). Figure 14.3 provides an adult BLS flow chart depicting the actions to be taken.

Table 14.1   The DRSABCD acronym

D	Danger	Check for danger. Before approaching the person, be sure it is safe to do so (the scene)
R	Response	If possible, approach the person from their feet; this prevents hyperextension of the neck from a responsive person
S	Shout for help	If you are on your own do not leave the person at this stage; shout for help
A	Airway	If the person is unresponsive open their airway using the head-tilt-chin lift method
B	Breathing	After opening the airway look, listen and feel for normal breathing for no more than 10 seconds
C	CPR/Circulation	If the person is not breathing, commence CPR (30 compressions and 2 breaths)
D	Defibrillation	If an automated external defibrillator (AED) is available this should be used alongside CPR

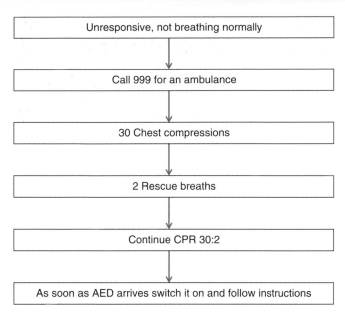

Figure 14.3   Adult basic life support flow chart. (Automatic external defibrillator (AED)).

Table 14.2   The AVPU scale for checking a response

		Explanation
A	Alert	Is the person alert, awake, talking, moving?
V	Verbal	Does the person respond to voice, such as direct questions or commands?
P	Place	The person does not respond when the rescuer places hands on the person's shoulders and gently shakes them, asking aloud '*Are you alright?*' Sometimes this is referred to as 'Pain' where gentle pressure is applied, e.g. to the ear lobe in order to elicit a response
U	Unresponsive	The person is unresponsive

The AVPU scale for checking a response

Table 14.2 outlines the AVPU scale.

Cardiopulmonary resuscitation (CPR)

Cardiopulmonary resuscitation (CPR) should be performed on a person who is not breathing normally and with no signs of life. CPR is an approach that combines chest compressions with rescue breaths with the intention of artificially circulating the blood and inflating the lungs.

1. Check for danger. Ensure that you are safe before you approach the person; check that there is no risk of fire or electrocution.
2. Check for a response. Shake the person's shoulders gently and shout 'Are you alright?'

3. If there is no response from the person, put them on their back. Warn others of the emergency situation and call for help by shouting 'I need some help here now'; you may also pull the emergency cord if you are in an environment where there is one.

4. If the person is in bed then remove the pillow from under them. Open the airway and observe for obstruction using a head tilt and chin lift movement. Place one hand on the forehead of the person and the fingers of your other hand under their chin and gently tilt the head back. If an injury to the person's cervical spine is suspected, perform a jaw thrust manoeuvre to open the airway. Do this by placing the ball of each palm on the person's cheek bones and two fingers from each hand under the angle of the mandible (jaw bone) before gently lifting the jaw forwards (Figure 14.4).

5. Use the look, listen and feel approach by placing your cheek next to the person's mouth and look down along their chest whilst feeling for a carotid pulse. Observe for any signs of life (breathing or movement), listen for breath sounds and feel for breaths on your cheek. After a maximum of ten seconds, you can confirm it is a cardiac arrest if there is no breathing and no signs of life or pulse. If the person has no signs of life, no pulse or when there is any doubt, start CPR immediately.

6. The rapid commencement of chest compressions is essential for positive outcomes, as is access to a defibrillator. If out of hospital call 999 or 112 for the emergency services. If in hospital, dial the cardiac arrest number and ask for the cardiac arrest team; you may ask the person who has come to your assistance to do this. Whoever makes the call must also request an automated external defibrillator (AED) if there is one is available.

7. Begin chest compressions on the non-responsive person immediately. Ensure you are able to get right over the centre of the person. Place your hands in the centre of the chest with the heel of one hand and the other one on top with your fingers interlocked and arms straight (Figure 14.5). Perform 30 chest compressions at a rate of between 100 and 120 per minute. Aim to depress the chest wall 5–6 cm ensuring adequate pressure is applied to compress the heart between the sternum (the breast bone) and the spinal column. Minimise interruptions to chest compressions (hands-off time).

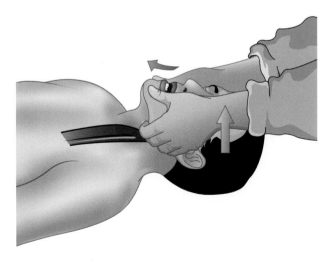

Figure 14.4   Jaw thrust.

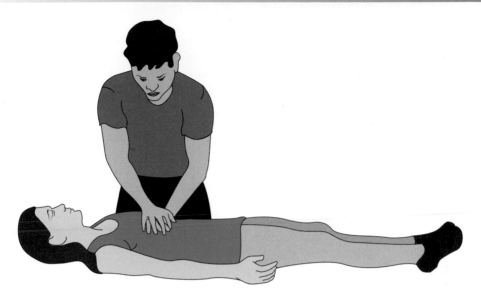

Figure 14.5   Chest compressions.

8. Provide two ventilations unless there are any reasons to avoid mouth-to-mouth or if you are unable to do it. If this is the case, perform continuous chest compressions at a rate of 100–120 per minute without stopping to give two breaths until help or airway equipment arrives. If you are in hospital or a care area where there is equipment available, provide ventilations using either a pocket mask or a bag valve mask (use local policy and procedure). If mouth-to-mouth is used to ventilate the person, you have to pinch the soft part of the nose closed, using the index finger and thumb; allow the mouth to open, maintain chin lift, take a normal breath, place the lips around, ensure a good seal is created. Blow steadily for approximately one second, take your mouth away and observe for the chest falling. Aim to provide two effective breaths over two seconds. If resistance is noted when attempting to inflate the lungs, the basic airway maintenance manoeuvres may need to be adjusted (head tilt and chin lift or jaw thrusts).

9. Continue with chest compressions and breaths at a ratio of 30:2. Performing chest compressions can be exhausting, so alternate regularly with any people who come to help you.

10. Do not stop chest compressions unless the person begins to show signs of regaining consciousness, coughs, opens their eyes or breathes normally.

11. If you have been trained in using the AED, when it arrives attach the pads to the person and follow the instructions, maintaining the safety of all those present. When the paramedics arrive (or the resuscitation team), they will begin advanced life support.

12. Observe the person using the Airway, Breathing, Circulation, Disability, Exposure (ABCDE) approach (Table 14.3), recording their physiological observations if able. You should document the resuscitation attempt.

13. After the BLS attempt seek support from your colleagues and manager so you are able to debrief.

Table 14.3   The ABCDE approach

		Explanation
A	Airway	Assess the airway by looking, listening and feeling. Observe the chest for movement and at the same time listen and/or feel for breath being expired from the mouth
B	Breathing	Assess breathing, looking, listening and feeling for signs of respiratory distress: • Sweating • Cyanosis (blueness) • The use of the accessory muscles of respiration Assess respiratory rate Assess the depth of each breath, the rhythm of breathing If the person is receiving oxygen note the amount being delivered Listen for noisy breathing, e.g. rattling or wheezing
C	Circulation	To assess circulation: • Look to see if hands are mottled, pale or cyanotic • Assess the limb temperature by touching the hands • Take a pulse – is it regular or irregular? Weak or strong? • Assess any wounds for signs of bleeding
D	Disability	Use the AVPU scale (see Table 14.2) to assess for response and consciousness
E	Exposure	This refers to exposing (or examining) the person, in order to assess for bleeding, signs of deterioration

Airway obstruction

There are many causes of airway obstruction. It can be due to the ingestion of a foreign body (including food), an allergic response, an asthma attack, a collection of blood, vomit or infections (e.g. laryngitis). An obstruction can result in minor or major breathing problems, and in some circumstances this can cause the person to become unconscious and unresponsive.

Airway obstruction can be partial or complete, and choking can cause either. The degree of difficulty in breathing will be determined by the cause of the obstruction. Signs and symptoms of an obstructed airway can include:

• collapse;
• grasping at the throat area;
• difficulty in breathing and speaking;
• abnormal breathing;
• stridor (noisy breathing);
• wheeze;
• difficulty in crying or making a noise;
• redness of the face;
• enlarged, bulging eyes and watering;
• displaying distress and fear.

For an adult you should:
• encourage the person to lean forwards and cough.

If the obstruction remains:

• administer a maximum of five sharp back blows (between the person's shoulder blades);
• administer a maximum of five abdominal thrusts.

Stop, look, respond 14.1

Pulses

In the diagram below locate the following pulse points:

1. Temporal
2. Carotid
3. Brachial
4. Femoral
5. Radial
6. Pedal

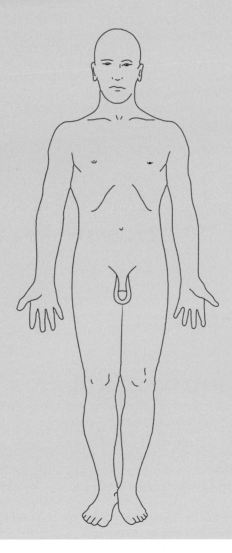

If the obstruction remains:

- Repeat the cycle two more times (three cycles in total).
- If after three cycles the obstruction remains, call for help, contact the emergency services and be ready to perform basic life support (CPR).

If there is a complete obstruction the person may show the above signs as well as a change in their skin colour, which may develop into a blue/grey tinge (cyanosis). The person will become progressively weaker and they will eventually become unconscious.

Training for managing airway obstruction should be provided by your employer.

Documentation

You may be required to complete your organisation's documentation concerning incidents and accidents should a person be involved in an incident or accident or if they become ill whilst in the health and social care setting; this will depend on your particular job role. Specific documentation will need to be completed. Noting this information in the incident/accident book can:

- help to alert managers and others to identify trends in incidents;
- help when managing health and safety risks;
- be used for reference in future first-aid needs assessments;
- be useful for any investigations should they arise.

You should ensure you adhere to agreed ways of working and make sure that you are aware of local policy and procedures.

Thinking cap 14.2

Incident and accident documentation

Identify where the incident and accident documentation in your organisation is located. What are you required to do should you have to make a record (document) of an incident or accident?

Automatic external defibrillators

When a high-energy electric shock is given to the heart, in some types of cardiac arrest this can restore a more stable rhythm. This is known as defibrillation and it is a vital life-saving step in the chain of survival.

Public access defibrillators (PADs) are often found in public areas such as shopping centres, gyms, bus and train stations, or community halls. PADs are briefcase-sized boxes that are mounted on the wall and contain a defibrillator. They are there for anyone to use on a person who is in cardiac arrest.

PADS are easy and safe to use. The machine provides clear spoken instructions. Once the defibrillator is open and in position, the defibrillator is able to detect the person's heart rhythm. It will not deliver a shock unless there is a need for one.

After a cardiac arrest has occurred, every minute without CPR and defibrillation can reduce a person's chance of survival by 10 per cent. When 999 is called, the operator will be able to tell the person making the call if there is access to a PAD close by. You should not interrupt chest compressions to get the PAD; if possible send someone else.

Chapter summary

- When a person has a cardiac arrest, BLS can be provided to help their chance of survival.
- BLS refers to the maintenance of a clear airway and support of breathing and circulation in cases of cardiac arrest.
- The best chance of a successful outcome is if chest compressions are started as soon as cardiac arrest has been diagnosed.
- The organisation for which you work should provide you with training for BLS and airway obstruction (choking).
- The Resuscitation Council United Kingdom provides a step-by-step guide for adult BLS reflecting up-to-date guidance.
- Attend regular updates of BLS to ensure that your knowledge and skills remain up to date.
- The acronym DRSABCD can be used when making a response to an unconscious person.
- Thirty compressions to two breaths are required.
- CPR should be performed on a person who is not breathing and shows no signs of life.
- The person should be observed using the Airway, Breathing, Circulation, Disability, Exposure approach.
- Airway obstruction can be partial or complete, and choking can cause either.
- You may be required to complete your organisation's documentation concerning incidents and accidents.
- A defibrillator is a device that gives a high-energy electric shock to the heart, which can, in some types of cardiac arrest, restore a more stable rhythm; this is known as defibrillation.

 ## Case scenario 14.1

Alan

Alan lives alone at home and receives support with the intention of maintaining his independence. A number of agencies provide services. Sunday is Alan's support worker and visits him on a daily basis to assist him with his personal hygiene and preparing his meals. Alan has recently been bereaved; he has just recovered from pneumonia.

Alan is walking to the toilet and he complains to Sunday of central, crushing, chest pain; Sunday sits him down. Alan say he can't breathe and the pain is now on the side of his face; he is clearly short of breath, is pale, feels cold and is clammy; he then collapses. Sunday, his carer, witnesses this and calls for an ambulance.

What should be Sunday's actions next, having called for an ambulance?

Resource file

British Red Cross
The British Red Cross helps people in crisis, whoever and wherever they are. It is part of a global voluntary network, responding to conflicts, natural disasters and individual emergencies.
http://www.redcross.org.uk

Resuscitation Council United Kingdom
The Resuscitation Council UK exists to promote high-quality, scientific, resuscitation guidelines that are applicable to everybody, contributing to the saving of life through education, training, research and collaboration.
https://www.resus.org.uk

St John Ambulance
The nation's leading first-aid charity. Campaigning to raise awareness of first aid and directly educate the public.
https://www.sja.org.uk

Chapter 15

Health and safety

Care certificate outcomes

1. Understand your own responsibilities, and the responsibilities of others, relating to health and safety in the work setting.
2. Understand risk assessment.
3. Move and assist safely.
4. Understand procedures for Stop, look, responding to accidents and sudden illness.
5. Understand medication and healthcare tasks.
6. Handle hazardous substances.
7. Promote fire safety.
8. Work securely.
9. Manage stress.

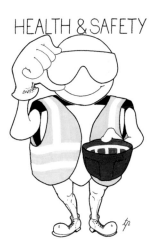

Fundamentals of Care: A Textbook for Health and Social Care Assistants, First Edition. Ian Peate.
© 2017 John Wiley & Sons Ltd. Published 2017 by John Wiley & Sons Ltd.

Take stock

Rate your current knowledge and skills prior to reading this chapter. Put a tick in the box that you think applies to you with regards to the standard being discussed:

Key:
I know this I have a good level of knowledge or skills regarding this aspect of the standard. I make use of the knowledge and skills identified on a regular basis, feeling confident in my ability and performance. I do not need a refresher.
Satisfactory My level of knowledge and standard of skills meet the criteria associated with the standard. I use the skills and knowledge from time to time. I might not always feel confident in my capability. I would benefit from a refresher.
I require a review I do not feel that I have the skills and/or the knowledge that would enable me to meet the standard in a confident and competent way. The knowledge and skills I used to have are no longer valid. I will require a refresher.
This is new to me I have never worked in a caring role before or I have never covered this topic before. I will need further training and development in this area.

Standard	Self-assessment			
Understand my responsibilities, and the responsibilities of others, with regards to health and safety in the workplace	☐ I know this	☐ Satisfactory	☐ I should review this	☐ This is new to me
Understand what risk assessment is	☐ I know this	☐ Satisfactory	☐ I should review this	☐ This is new to me
Describe how to move and assist safely	☐ I know this	☐ Satisfactory	☐ I should review this	☐ This is new to me
Outline the procedures for Stop, look, responding to accidents and sudden illness	☐ I know this	☐ Satisfactory	☐ I should review this	☐ This is new to me
Provide an understanding of medication and healthcare tasks	☐ I know this	☐ Satisfactory	☐ I should review this	☐ This is new to me
Understand safe ways in handling hazardous substances	☐ I know this	☐ Satisfactory	☐ I should review this	☐ This is new to me
Promote fire safety	☐ I know this	☐ Satisfactory	☐ I should review this	☐ This is new to me
Understand ways to work safely	☐ I know this	☐ Satisfactory	☐ I should review this	☐ This is new to me
Describe ways in which stress can be managed	☐ I know this	☐ Satisfactory	☐ I should review this	☐ This is new to me

Introduction

Everyone in the workplace, all of us, from the employer to the newest worker, have different but nevertheless important duties to perform in order to keep the workplace safe.

Employers have the greatest responsibility in the workplace and because of this they have the most authority regarding health and safety issues. However, it is important for your own safety that you understand everyone's health and safety duties, including yours. A key duty of any employer is to provide you with specific information and instructions about how to stay safe whilst performing your duties.

 Stop, look, respond 15.1

Harm

Who do you think is more likely to get hurt or sick whilst at work?

- New and young workers

or

- experienced workers?

New and young workers are more likely to get hurt during their first month on the job than at any other time. That is because often they are not told about or do not understand the hazards of the job. They do not know what to expect from their employer, their supervisor and themselves. Sometimes they are not sure what questions to ask and sometimes they do not even know whom to ask.

The law

There are a number of laws that cover or address the health and safety of people at work and those affected by work activities including people who receive care and support services.

Table 15.1 provides an overview of some of those pieces of legislation that provide statutory guidance affecting people in the workplace. Policies related to health and safety at work are usually derived from legislation. Health and safety rules and guidance aim to reduce the risk of hazards to a worker's physical and emotional wellbeing whilst at work. All policies and procedures inform everyone how to do something or what must be in place to ensure that all people are safe.

Health and safety policies

Policies and procedures work together; they clarify what your organisation wants and how you should go about doing it. Policies are clear, simple statements providing a set of guiding principles to help with decision making. Procedures describe how each policy will be put into action. Policies must give clear instructions so that everyone is kept safe and nobody is harmed as a result of the work that is being carried out. You have a responsibility to familiarise yourself with health and safety policies and procedures in your own workplace.

Stop, look, respond 15.2

Policies and procedures

Where can you locate polices in your workplace regarding:

- Smoking in the workplace?
- The use of mobile phones?
- Alcohol consumption in the workplace?
- Drug use/substance abuse?
- Lone working/home care working?
- Needle-stick injury?
- The use of computers?

What do your own organisation's procedures say about:

- The storage and administration of oxygen?
- How to offer personal care?
- What to do in the event of an injury occurring?
- What to do if a person refuses care or support?
- How to dispose of sharps?
- How to make known your concerns if you think a person is at risk of abuse?

Health and safety policies produced by employers set out how they aim to protect all of those who are affected by their business, for example their employees, visitors, contractors and those people who access the services that they provide. Health and safety legislation applies even when the employee works in the private homes of those you offer care to or provide support to. Your manager will be able to inform you about policies that are in place to provide you with support regarding your health, safety and wellbeing whilst at work.

Hazards in the workplace

You have the right to refuse to do unsafe work if you have reason to believe that it might put you or a fellow worker in danger. A hazard can be considered as anything in the workplace that could harm you or those with whom you work.

There is a hazard at the core of every work-related death, injury or sickness. A hazard can take many forms. Sometimes more than one hazard can combine to make an even bigger hazard. It is important that you know about the hazards in your workplace prior to your starting work.

Thinking cap 15.1

Hazards at work

Think about the people you know. Do you know anyone who has been hurt or killed whilst at work? What was the hazard at the root of it? How did you feel about it? How did it affect the other person's family?

Table 15.1   Elements of legislation associated with health and safety at work

Element of legislation	Description
Health and Safety at Work Act 1974	A general Act detailing how employers have a legal duty to assess all risks to the health and safety of employees. If the risk assessment shows that it is not possible for the work to be done safely, then other arrangements must be put in place
Management of Health and Safety at Work Regulations 1999	Concerns how health and safety is managed within a care workplace, including risk assessment, training and ensuring that employees have access to the information they need
Manual Handling Operations Regulations 1992	Offers information and training on lifting and handling. Addresses the transporting or supporting of any load and how to perform this safely and prevent injury
Lifting Operations and Lifting Equipment Regulations 1998	Also known as LOLER, these regulations require that all equipment used for lifting is fit for purpose, appropriate for the task, suitably marked and, in many cases, subject to statutory periodic checks through examination
Provision and Use of Work Equipment Regulations 1998	Also known as PUWER, this covers all work equipment from office furniture through to complex machinery and company cars; it is also applicable if a company allows a worker to use their own equipment in the workplace and how this is to be used safely
Control of Substances Hazardous to Health Regulations 1999	Information and training on any chemicals used under the Control of Substances Hazardous to Health (COSHH). The regulations require employers to control substances that are hazardous to health
The Regulatory Reform (Fire Safety) Order 2005	Details how every workplace must prevent/protect against fire. The Order covers general fire precautions and other fire safety duties that are needed to protect relevant persons in case of fire in and around most premises. Fire precautions are required to be put in place where necessary and to the extent that it is reasonable and practicable in the circumstances of the case
Reporting of Injuries, Diseases and Dangerous Occurrences Regulations 1995	More commonly known as RIDDOR. Employers have to report to the enforcing authorities certain accidents suffered by employees, including incidents of violence. Accident and incident reporting are an important part of work in any health or social care workplace
Facilities for First Aid Under the Health and Safety (First Aid) Regulations 1981	Sets out the essential aspects of first aid that employers have to address. Employers must provide adequate and appropriate equipment, ensuring also that employees receive immediate attention if they are injured or taken ill at work
Personal Protective Equipment at Work Regulations 1992	Personal Protective Equipment (PPE) also includes clothing. The employers must provide PPE to staff whenever health and safety risks are not adequately protected by other means. The employee has a duty to use PPE in accordance with training and instruction given by their employer

Workplace hazards

There are a number of common workplace hazards (Figure 15.1).

Safety hazards

These are the most common type of hazards and can present in any workplace environment at one time or another. They include unsafe conditions that could result in injury or death, for example:

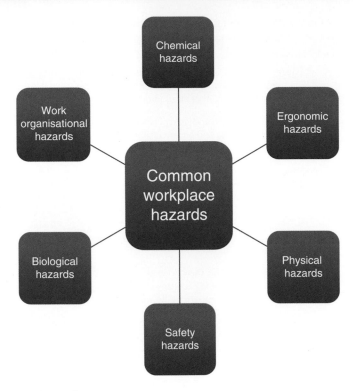

Figure 15.1   Workplace hazards.

- spills on the floor;
- tripping hazards such as cords trailing across the floor;
- rugs that slip;
- unguarded machinery and machinery with moving parts;
- electrical hazards;
- working in confined spaces;
- machinery-related hazards (medical equipment).

Biological hazards

Biological hazards are associated with working with people and infectious materials. Working in nursing homes, residential care facilities, a person's home, hospitals and so on could expose the health and care worker to biological hazards. Exposure to the following can prove hazardous:

- blood, blood products;
- body fluids;
- bacteria;
- viruses;
- fungi.

Chemical hazards

Any chemical that has the ability to cause harm is called a hazardous or dangerous chemical. It is impossible to avoid being exposed to chemicals; every day in our homes, schools or shops there are hundreds of different types of chemicals that we are exposed to.

Chemical hazards are present when health or social care workers are exposed to any chemical preparation in the workplace; this can be in any form, whether liquid, solid or gas. Some people are more sensitive to certain chemicals than others, and this may cause illness, breathing problems or skin irritations. The following can cause illness and disease:

- anaesthetic and medical gases;
- solvents;
- vapours and fumes;
- flammable materials;
- disinfectants;
- bleach;
- pharmaceutical substances;
- cytotoxic drugs;
- laboratory chemicals.

Physical hazards

An external factor that can harm the body is known as a physical hazard, even though the person may not necessarily touch it. These include:

- radiation;
- excessive exposure to sunlight/ultraviolet rays;
- extremes of temperature;
- exposure to constant loud noise;
- constant light or dark (dim) environments.

Ergonomic exposure

This is associated with the type of work a person does, and concerns body positions or working conditions that put a constant strain on the body. Long-term exposure can result in serious and chronic illness with reduced mobility. Ergonomic exposure includes:

- improperly adjusted workstations and chairs;
- frequent lifting;
- poor posture;
- awkward, repetitive movements;
- repeating the same movement over and over;
- having to use too much force, particularly if this needs to be done frequently.

Work organisation hazards

These hazards or stressors can have short- or long-term effects. They are related to workplace issues, such as workload and exposure to unpleasant occurrences (heard or seen), for example:

- excessive workload demands;
- not having any control over work;
- the potential (or actual) exposure to workplace violence;
- intensity or pace of work;
- lack of flexibility;
- lack of social support or relations;
- dealing with crises;
- seeing or hearing unpleasant incidents.

Thinking cap 15.2

Minimising risks

Think about your day at work. Now think about the potential workplace hazards that exist. Did you encounter any of them at work? How might you minimise the risks and potential harm associated with them?

Working with hazardous substances

Hazardous substances can be present in the air, water and the food we eat. At work the main routes of exposure are through:

- inhalation (breathing in the chemical);
- inoculation (i.e. needle-stick injury);
- absorption (through the skin or a splash in the eye);
- ingestion (via contaminated food or hands).

You should read the hazard information that can be found on the label of all products that you use. This will provide you with information about the hazards associated with use and may help to keep you and other people safe. You must always ensure that you work in agreed ways to protect your own health and wellbeing as well as those of the people around you.

The place where you work must have a secure area designated solely for the storage of hazardous substances. There are some hazardous substances that should only be handled when you are wearing PPE. Policies and procedures set out when PPE should be worn, and these will normally include the handling of clinical waste and certain chemicals.

Reporting health and safety hazards

Your employer is responsible for carrying out risk assessments to identify the actions that need to be taken to protect staff and visitors from hazards. Where there are more than five people in the organisation, the assessment should be recorded. It is not just the employer's responsibility to find hazards in the workplace. Everybody has a part to play in reducing risks, and it is important that you know what to do if you identify a hazard.

The workplace will become a safer place for you and others when people are aware of any potential hazards. If you see something that you think may be hazardous in the workplace, report it to your manager immediately.

If you are an employee or a member of the public and you think the health and safety law is being broken, or that minimum standards are being ignored within the workplace, you can try to resolve the concern yourself by:

- Speaking to the employer or the person in charge to try to resolve the issue.
- Contacting your work/safety representative, or your trade union, who can try to resolve the issue for you.

If the matter is not satisfactorily resolved, you can raise it with the relevant enforcing authority, for example the Health and Safety Executive (the UK regulator for health and safety in the workplace), or your local authority.

Thinking cap 15.3

Making concerns known

What mechanisms are in place in your workplace that allow you to report or make known health and safety concerns? Is there any accident/incident book/form that has to be completed?

Risk assessment

A risk assessment is the process of defining what hazards exist or might exist in the workplace that are likely to cause harm to employees and visitors. Some areas where hazards are likely to be identified include electrical safety, fire safety, manual handling or hazardous substances. Less obvious dangers also exist, and the employer must consider things such as the risk of repetitive strain injuries or work-related stress.

When a risk assessment is undertaken this can help to identify any actual or potential hazards. A risk assessment is a legal requirement (Management of Health and Safety at Work Regulations 1999); it can also help to provide clear guidance and information on how to keep people safe and to prevent danger, harm and accidents. The assessment will identify hazards in the workplace, assess the degree of risk, and determine measures or procedures to be put in place in order to reduce the identified risk.

A risk assessment is not about generating large amounts of paperwork; it is more about identifying sensible measures to control the risks in the workplace. Consideration should be given to how accidents and ill health might occur and concentrate on real risks, those that are more probable and that will cause the most harm. The risk is the possibility, high or low, that a person could be harmed by hazards, along with an idea of how serious the harm could be.

A basic risk assessment should be simple to conduct and is guided by a process that includes:

- Looking for and making a list of the risks to health and safety.
- Deciding who may be harmed and how.
- Checking that protective measures are efficient.
- Assessing the risks that arise from the hazards and determining if current precautions are satisfactory.
- Recording the findings.
- Re-evaluating the assessment from time to time and amending it when needed.

Figure 15.2 outlines the five steps associated with risk assessment.

Accidents and incidents

Injuries, incidents and accidents can and do occur in the workplace, both to staff and to those for whom you care or offer support, despite risk assessments and hazards identified. In those workplaces where there are more significant health and safety risks there is a need for staff to receive training as first-aiders. If you have not attended any first-aid training you should not carry out any form of first aid, but must seek help immediately. Attempting first aid without any specialist training could make the injury or the person's condition worse. For many health and care workers first aid is an important aspect of their induction programme.

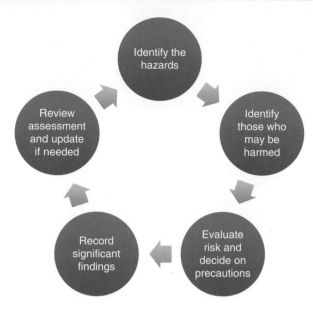

Figure 15.2   The five steps associated with a risk assessment.

Table 15.2   What to do in emergency situations

- Stay calm and call for help by shouting, phoning or finding someone
- Observe the person, listen to what they are saying, try to determine what has happened, reassure them, but do not move the person unless it is absolutely necessary for safety
- Remain with the injured or sick person until assistance arrives, observing and making a note of any changes in their condition. Do this as you will be required to inform relevant medical staff or others of what you have seen
- Do as little as you need to do in order to keep the person stable and alive until qualified help arrives
- Document all activity in a full report and adhere to the agreed ways of working when informing carers or family members who need to know
- You may wish to reflect on the activity with other people with whom you work

You have to ensure that the safety of the individuals and everyone else who may be involved in any accident or incident is protected. Your workplace will have health and safety procedures in place that will describe what to do in an emergency; ensure that you are familiar with these. Being familiar with the person's care plan will inform you if that person is known to have a condition that may lead to sudden illness, as well as describing the ways in which you should respond. Table 15.2 outlines what you should do in emergency situations.

Medicines

The people who use care services should be able to expect that they will receive their medication in a safe and timely manner. Medication training is usually an important aspect of a health or social worker's induction. Those who have not undertaken this training will not be able to administer medication in a residential care home or care agency registered with the Care Quality Commission.

The elements of medication training will vary as each care organisation will have different needs, and as such there is no approved list of what should be covered as part of medication training. Training has to be delivered by an appropriately trained individual. E-learning and videos can contribute to training but they should not be seen as the main delivery method.

Some people you support may require your help to store and take their medication correctly, whereas others will be able to manage their own medication safely. Encouraging those who can manage their own medication safely can promote their independence. In each person's care or support plan there will be information about the type of support the person needs. You should be aware of the agreed ways of working in your organisation and the policies and procedures relating to medication management.

Unless it is a part of your role and until you have completed and satisfactorily passed the appropriate training you must not remind, assist or provide people with their medication. This will include any inhaled medications, medications that need to be swallowed, the application of any medical creams/ointments, drops, or prompting or helping with injections. Generally you should not undertake any actions that are not described in the person's care or support plan.

Moving, handling and assisting

It is more than likely that all care workers will be required to assist and move somebody for whom they are providing care. You will also be moving and handling objects. There is an expectation that appropriate training will be provided by the employer in order to perform this activity safely and effectively.

Prior to undertaking any assisting and moving activities, and in order to protect the person using the service, training should have been provided and completed. Training can include hands-on practical demonstrations along with (but not restricted to) workbooks and/or e-learning. Safe and effective assisting and moving training can help you (and if needed, others who are assisting you) to help people who need:

- to get into or out of a bed, to turn over in a bed, sit up in a bed;
- assistance with hygiene needs, such as having a bath, taking a shower;
- to use the toilet/commode;
- to sit in a chair;
- to stand up, mobilise, get up from the floor after falling;
- to get in and out of a vehicle.

You may be required to use equipment, for example hoists, assisted beds and lifts, to move people and objects in a safe way. The equipment that you will be required to use will come with instructions for safe use; make yourself familiar with these.

There are laws that apply to activities that involve lifting, putting down, pushing, pulling, carrying or moving by hand or bodily force. You and your employer are required to abide by those laws. You must have appropriate training before using any equipment so that you do not injure yourself or the person you are caring for or offering support to. The agreed ways for undertaking moving, handling and assisted tasks will be detailed in local policies and procedures, and there will also be details in the person's individual care plan.

Fire safety awareness

The employer has to ensure that people who provide fire safety training have the appropriate qualifications, experience or background to deliver the training to a satisfactory standard.

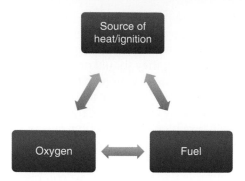

Figure 15.3   Components required to support a fire.

Once a fire starts it can grow very quickly and spread from one source of fuel to another. As it grows, the amount of heat given off increases and this in turn can cause other fuels to self-ignite. Three things are needed for a fire to start (Figure 15.3):

1. A source of heat/ignition
2. Fuel
3. Oxygen

If any one of the three components described in Figure 15.3 is missing a fire cannot start. Taking steps to avoid these three things coming together and identifying hazards will therefore reduce the likelihood of a fire occurring.

Potential sources of ignition

The potential ignition sources in the workplace can be identified by looking for possible sources of heat that could get hot enough to ignite the material in the workplace. These sources of heat could include:

- arson;
- smokers' materials;
- naked flames;
- cooking;
- electrical sparks/faulty electrical appliances.

There are indicators of 'near misses', for example scorch marks on furniture or fittings, discoloured or charred electrical plugs and sockets, or cigarette burns. These can help you to identify hazards that you may not otherwise be aware of.

 Thinking cap 15.4

Near misses

Look around the area where you work and determine if there are any indicators of 'near misses'.

Identifying sources of fuel

Anything that can burn is fuel for a fire. You need to be alert to the things that will burn reasonably easily and are in sufficient quantity to provide fuel for a fire or cause it to spread to another fuel source. Some of the most common 'fuels' found in the workplace are:

- paper and card;
- plastics, rubber and foam such as polystyrene, e.g. the foam used in upholstered furniture and mattresses;
- flammable gases;
- textiles;
- loose packaging material.

Identifying sources of oxygen

The air surrounding us is the main source of oxygen for a fire. In an enclosed building this is provided by the ventilation system or through open windows required for ventilation.

Additional sources of oxygen can be found in materials used or stored in the workplace or in a person's home, such as oxygen supplies from chamber storage and piped systems, for example oxygen used for healthcare purposes.

In reducing risk the aim is to decrease or minimise the sources of ignition and to minimise the potential fuel for a fire.

Stop, look, respond 15.3

Fire

Clearly describe the actions you need to take if you discover a fire in the building.

_____

_____

_____

_____

_____

_____

_____

_____

The place where you work will have its own procedures in place and actions that need to be taken in the event of a fire. You must ensure that you are familiar with these procedures. If you work in a person's home find out where the escape routes are and, with your manager, decide on what would need to be done in case of a fire.

Stop, look, respond 15.4

Emergencies

Describe what you should do if the following emergencies occurred in the place where you work:

- Fire
- Security alert
- Serious accident in your work area
- Minor accident, where someone needs first aid
- Major incident, where someone has an anaphylactic reaction
- A chemical spill

Think about:

- Who you need to communicate with
- Your role in offering assistance
- What you should do if you are first on the scene
- The role you play in reporting the incident

Working safely

Health and social care staff should be able to attend their work without fear of violence, abuse or harassment from patients, their relatives or others. In the majority of cases, patients and their relatives will be appreciative towards those who treat them or offer them support, but some people may be abusive or violent towards staff.

Concerns about violent conduct of those who use services or visitors towards health and social care staff have encouraged a zero tolerance policy within the NHS. The place where you work will have procedures in place to address your security whilst at work. You can also help to ensure your own safety; for example:

- Ensure any visitors sign a visitors book.
- Challenge any strangers who should not have access to the premises.
- Ensure you have with you any personal alarm system you have been issued with.
- Check the identity of individuals in person or those who telephone seeking information.

If you work in unsafe ways, in ways that have not been agreed with your employer and without suitable training, this can mean that you will be putting yourself, the people you care for and support, and others at risk of injury.

Managing stress

Work-related stress can be the response when people are exposed to excessive pressures or other types of demands that are placed upon them in their job. A poor match between the worker and the work, conflicts between roles at work and outside of it, and not having a reasonable degree of control over work and life balance can all be causes of stress. There are a multitude of stressors.

Stop, look, respond 15.5

Health and safety training updates

You must regularly update your training associated with health and safety.

Make notes in the list below concerning updates with regards to health and safety training, and make a note of your next date for a training update. You may need to seek assistance from your manager to complete this. Other training activity may be provided to you that is specifically related to your place of work and the role you are undertaking.

Training activity	Frequency of update (date of your next update)
First aid	
Fire safety	
Food hygiene	
Medication	
Infection prevention and control	
Moving and handling	
Protection of vulnerable people	
COSHH	
Dignified care and responsibility training	
Basic life support	
Other	
Other	

Stress may cause changes in those experiencing it. In some instances there are clear signs that a person is experiencing stress at work. If these can be identified early then action can be taken before this becomes a problem.

The changes may only be noticeable to the person who is experiencing the stress. Therefore it is important for you to pay attention to how you are feeling and try to identify any potential issues you may have as early as possible, taking positive action to address them. For example, discuss the matter with a line manager, talk to staff in the occupational health department or with your own GP.

The events and situations that can activate or exacerbate stress will differ from person to person. Some people can take on pressures and demands prior to displaying signs of stress, whereas others may not be able to take as much pressure or demands.

Stress is not a disease; however, if stress is excessive and goes on for some time, it can lead to psychological and physical ill health. Stress reveals itself in many ways, impacting on an individual physically and psychologically and affecting a number of bodily functions (Figure 15.4).

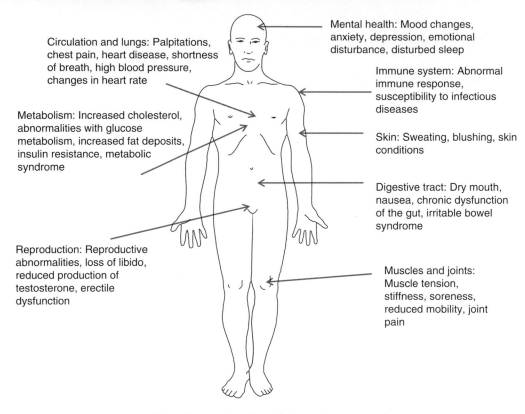

Figure 15.4   Some aspects of the physical and psychological impact of stress.

Signs of stress in a group may include:

- disagreements and disaffection within the group;
- increase in staff renewal rate;
- increase in complaints and grievances amongst staff;
- increased sickness absence rates;
- increased accounts and reporting of stress;
- challenges in attracting new staff;
- poor performance;
- customer dissatisfaction or complaints.

Employees have a duty to be responsible for their own health and safety at work and that of those around them with regards to stress. Employees should be encouraged to:

- Become knowledgeable about stress, ensuring they are aware of and understand policies and procedures.
- Come to terms with their own feelings so they know when they are feeling stressed.
- Develop effective behavioural skills such as assertiveness and time management, which can reduce the stress they are feeling.
- Establish a support network.
- Develop a lifestyle that protects against stress.

Thinking cap 15.5

Stress

How do you manage stress?

All of us manage and respond to the various stressors encountered in different ways, and the ways in which we react and the strategies we employ for responding to them will differ.

Chapter summary

- There are several aspects of legislation that relate to health and safety.
- Health and safety in the workplace is everyone's responsibility, both employers and employees.
- There are many tasks/activities that you undertake as part of your work that you will require special training for.
- There are a number of specific tasks/activities that you are not allowed to carry out until you have received specific training for them and you have been deemed competent, for example the management of medications.
- You must be aware of your employer's agreed ways of working with regards to certain health- and social care-related tasks.
- The workplace contains a number of hazards that could cause harm to you or the people you care for or offer support to. Where possible you should be alert to these hazards.
- A health and safety risk assessment can help to identify hazards and provide solutions with the aim of minimising risk and harm.
- You are required to understand procedures for responding to accidents and sudden illness, but you must only act within the sphere of your competence.
- In the majority of cases, patients and their relatives will be appreciative towards those who treat them or offer them support.
- Health and social care staff should be able to attend their work without fear of violence, abuse or harassment from patients, their relatives or others.
- Workplace stress can have a negative impact on a person from physiological, behavioural and psychological perspectives.
- Events and situations that can activate or exacerbate stress differ from person to person.
- We all manage and respond to the various stressors in different ways.

Case scenario 15.1

The new care home

A newly built care home had received reports from the care staff that the carpets in the home made the mobile patient hoist far too difficult to manoeuvre. As a result of this the staff stopped using the hoists, putting them and the people they provided care to at risk.

A risk assessment was undertaken and the carers identified that the carpets were an important risk factor when attempting to move the hoist. When a patient was in the hoist, staff observed that the wheels sank into the carpet and this made it difficult to move. The wheels of the hoist were made from rubber, which is appropriate for floors that are smooth and/or hard.

The managers of the home contacted the supplier. The supplier responded and said it was possible to change the wheels of the hoist to a type that was more suited for use on carpets; the wheel material was changed to polyurethane. The force required to manoeuvre using the hoist with the polyurethane wheels was reduced by nearly half as a result of the new wheels. The care staff are now using the hoist when needed for moving patients.

Can you think of any other solutions to the problem?

 Resource file

Health and Safety Executive
The Health and Safety Executive aims to reduce work-related deaths, injuries and ill health.
http://www.hse.gov.uk

Workplace Health and Safety Standards
A set of standards developed with the support of the Health and Safety Executive pulling together legal requirements and guidance to help organisations comply with legislation.
http://www.nhsemployers.org/~/media/Employers/Publications/workplace-health-safety-standards.pdf

Health, Safety and Wellbeing Partnership Group
The overall purpose of the Health, Safety and Wellbeing Partnership Group is to raise standards of workplace health, safety and wellbeing in healthcare organisations, to promote a safer working environment for all healthcare staff and to promote best practice across both the NHS and the independent sector.
http://www.nhsemployers.org/your-workforce/pay-and-reward/national-negotiations/nhs-staff-council/health-safety-and-wellbeing-partnership-group-hswpg

Chapter 16
Handling information

Care certificate outcomes

1. Handle information.

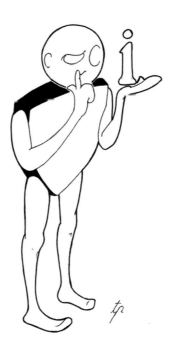

Fundamentals of Care: A Textbook for Health and Social Care Assistants, First Edition. Ian Peate.
© 2017 John Wiley & Sons Ltd. Published 2017 by John Wiley & Sons Ltd.

Take stock

Rate your current knowledge and skills prior to reading this chapter. Put a tick in the box that you think applies to you with regards to the standard being discussed:

Key:
I know this I have a good level of knowledge or skills regarding this aspect of the standard. I make use of the knowledge and skills identified on a regular basis, feeling confident in my ability and performance. I do not need a refresher.
Satisfactory My level of knowledge and standard of skills meet the criteria associated with the standard. I use the skills and knowledge from time to time. I might not always feel confident in my capability. I would benefit from a refresher.
I require a review I do not feel that I have the skills and/or the knowledge that would enable me to meet the standard in a confident and competent way. The knowledge and skills I used to have are no longer valid. I will require a refresher.
This is new to me I have never worked in a caring role before or I have never covered this topic before. I will need further training and development in this area.

Standard	Self-assessment			
Describe the agreed ways of working and legislation regarding the recording, storing and sharing of information	☐ I know this	☐ Satisfactory	☐ I should review this	☐ This is new to me
Explain why it is important to have secure systems for recording, storing and sharing information	☐ I know this	☐ Satisfactory	☐ I should review this	☐ This is new to me
Describe how to keep records that are up to date, complete, accurate and legible	☐ I know this	☐ Satisfactory	☐ I should review this	☐ This is new to me
Explain how, and to whom, to report if you become aware that agreed ways of working have not been followed	☐ I know this	☐ Satisfactory	☐ I should review this	☐ This is new to me

Introduction

It is important to have secure systems for recording and storing information in order to safeguard and protect each individual's human rights. This is known as information governance, and is to do with the way an organisation processes or handles information. It addresses personal information, for example the personal information relating to the people you offer care or support to, as well as information about employees and corporate information, including financial and accounting records. As part of duty of care the health and social care worker has a duty of confidentiality with respect to the way information is shared and stored as well as the way it is recorded.

The information gathered must be collected carefully, ensuring it is accurate; this also applies to the ways in which it is retained, be this manually or electronically. Whichever system is used it must be secure. The health and social care worker has to be aware of issues that surround the way in which information is accessed and with whom they share information, particularly in relation to freedom of information and the principle of confidentiality.

There are policies and procedures in your workplace for agreed ways of working including those related to interagency as well as multi-agency and integrated working. These policies and procedures set out your roles and responsibilities and will also refer to the need for staff training concerning the handling of information.

You must follow procedures and codes of practice for handling information, whilst seeking permission from the appropriate person to access records where and when needed. Confidentiality of information is a key element of maintaining dignity for those people who use health and social care services.

Personal information should be safeguarded. If personal information is lost, stolen or used inappropriately this can be used for illegal purposes. Filing cabinets should be locked when unattended. Computers should have password protection to limit access to files containing information about staff and those who use services. More sensitive information will require additional safeguards. The best safeguard is to not collect or keep more information than is needed; this way there is less risk of this information being misused.

Thinking cap 16.1

Personal information

Think about the personal information that organisations hold about you. Imagine that information was disclosed (deliberately or unintentionally) to others. What do you think they might be able to do with your personal information?

Key legislation

There are several elements of law (legislation) that control the ways in which information is handled. All public and private organisations have a legal duty to protect any personal information that they hold. Public bodies are also required to provide public access to official information.

Laws have been enacted to control the use of personal information; including information that has been stored in computer databases. This ensures that the individual's rights to confidentiality and an organisation's need to use it are balanced.

Data Protection Act 1998

The Data Protection Act covers the processing of personal data on a computer or an organised paper filing system. The Act controls the way information is handled and gives legal rights to people who have information stored about them.

As more and more personal information is stored and processed on computers there is always a danger that the information could be misused or get into the wrong hands. Concerns arise around who might access this information, how accurate the information is, could the information be easily copied, and has the information stored about the person been given with the person's knowledge or permission.

Some data and information stored about a person on a computer are personal and have to be kept confidential. Personal data refer to information concerning an identified or identifiable living individual, which is processed automatically (through a computer) or recorded manually as part of a filing system or part of an accessible record. The data will include records such as a health record or social service file. Processing includes anything done in relation to the data, such as collecting it, holding it, disclosing it and destroying it.

If someone who is not entitled to see these details accesses them without permission it is unauthorised access. The Data Protection Act sets up rules to prevent this happening.

When there is a risk of harm to other people, then there are some limits on confidentiality – for example, if there are issues concerning safeguarding. A data controller is a person or company that collects and keeps data about people; they decide how and why personal data are processed. The eight data protection principles that are central to the Act are given in Table 16.1.

Table 16.1   The eight data protection principles

Personal details:
1. Must be collected and used fairly and inside the law
2. Must only be held and used for the reasons given to the Information Commissioner (the person responsible for enforcing the act)
3. Can only be used for those registered purposes and only be disclosed to those people mentioned in the register entry. They cannot be given away or sold unless the person said they could be to begin with
4. The information held must be adequate, relevant and not excessive when compared with the purpose stated in the register. There must be enough detail but not too much for the intended use
5. Must be accurate and be kept up to date. There is a duty to keep them up to date, for example to change an address when a person moves
6. Must not be kept longer than is necessary for the registered purpose. It is acceptable to keep information for a certain length of time but not indefinitely
7. Must be kept safe and secure, including keeping the information backed up and away from any unauthorised access. It is wrong to leave personal data open to be viewed by just anyone
8. May not be transferred outside of the European Economic Area unless the country that the data is being sent to has a suitable data protection law

Stop, look, respond 16.1

Personal information

Your organisation will have a reasonable purpose, or a good reason, for collecting personal information from staff and the people they provide services to.

Create a list of your organisation's purposes for collecting personal information.

In your opinion, is there any personal information that your organisation collects for no apparent good reason? If you cannot link the information to a purpose, consider whether they should be collecting it. Organisations should collect only what they reasonably need.

The Freedom of Information Act 2000

This Act provides public access to information held by public authorities. Public authorities are required to publish certain information about their activities and members of the public are permitted to request information from public authorities.

The Act includes any recorded information that is held by a public authority. Public authorities include government departments, local authorities, the NHS (including dentists and GP surgeries), state schools, universities and police forces and prisons. The Act does not, for example, cover some charities that receive grants and certain private sector organisations that perform public functions. Recorded information includes:

- printed documents;
- computer files;
- letters;
- emails;
- photographs;
- sound or video recordings.

The Act does not give people access to their own personal data (information about themselves), for example their health or social records. If a member of the public wants to see information that a public authority holds about them, they have to make a subject access request under the Data Protection Act 1998. A public authority may determine that the information it holds is covered by a qualified exemption or exception, in which case it must apply the public interest test. In essence the public authority has to identify the reason why release of the information is not in the public interest.

A person has the right to make a subject access request, and if this is granted it can include documents, reports and emails that have been written between two co-workers. Anything that is added to any record must be accurate and suitable to be viewed by those it concerns.

Stop, look, respond 16.2

Management and safety of personal information

In your organisation who takes the overall lead with regards to the management and safety of information? Who would you contact if you have questions with regards to the management and safety of personal information (yours or the people who use your services)?

The electronic patient record

This is sometimes called the electronic medical record or the electronic health record; the terms are often used interchangeably.

Essentially these types of record are a way of viewing a person's medical or social care record via a computerised interface, a digital version of the person's paper record. The electronic record is a real-time, person-centred record that makes information available instantly and securely to authorised users; the information moves with the person. Health and social care information can be created and managed by authorised providers in a digital format with the capability of being shared with other providers across more than one health and or social care organisation, including,

221

for example, laboratories, health and social care specialists, medical imaging facilities, pharmacies and emergency facilities. These records contain information from all involved in a person's health and social care. The electronic record means that the person's information is available without having to wait for the paper record to be brought or found.

Stop, look, respond 16.3

The electronic record

Complete the list below:

Advantages of the electronic record	Disadvantages of the electronic record

Confidentiality is protected through the use of security measures for handling information. Access to a person's electronic record is only possible if the health or social care worker has a smartcard with a PIN number and a genuine relationship with the person. Each time a person's information is accessed, an electronic record of this is made.

In order to access and manage health and social care information safely your employer will have agreed ways of working in place to protect that information; they have a duty to ensure that this is in place. Organisations will have a computer firewall and password protection in place to restrict access to electronic information. Passwords should never be shared and should only be used by those who have permission to access the information. Where paper-based systems are in use there will also be guidelines available, for example where records are kept, who has access to them, and who contributes to them.

Agreed ways of working will also be evident even when you are providing care and support to a person in their own home. You will need to know what records there are and where they are to be kept.

In care plans or any other documents (electronic or paper) that you use it is essential that you include all details of the agreed care (provided and omitted), as well as ensuring that your writing is neat and legible and that the meaning is clear. Care plans are an essential record of a person's unique needs and choices and include an assessment of risks. A care plan is an important tool in effective communication between those who are involved in providing care and support. You should avoid using jargon and ensure that the information you are providing is factual and not based on opinion. Care plans should be checked regularly to ensure they are fit for purpose and are a true reflection of the needs or support the person requires.

The principles of good record keeping can be found in Table 16.2.

Thinking cap 16.2

Care plans

In your place of work how often are care plans updated? Who has responsibility for this?

Table 16.2   The principles of good record keeping

- You should only write in records (electronic or paper) if you have permission to do so and you are competent to do so
- Use handwriting that is legible
- Any entry to records should be signed. In the case of written records, your name and job title should be printed alongside the first entry
- You should put the date and time on all records. This should be in real time and chronological order and be as close to the actual time as possible. You must adhere to local policy
- Records should be accurate and clear
- Records should be factual; do not include unnecessary abbreviations, jargon, meaningless phrases or irrelevant speculation
- You should adhere to local policy or seek advice in deciding what is relevant and what should be recorded
- You should record details of any assessments and reviews undertaken as well as details of information given about care and treatment
- Records should identify any risks or problems that have developed and show the action taken to deal with them
- You must not alter or destroy any records without being authorised to do so
- Should you need to alter your own records, you must give your name and job title and sign and date the original documentation. Make sure that alterations made and the original record, are clear and auditable
- The language that you use should be easily understood by the people in your care
- Records should be readable when photocopied or scanned
- You should not use coded expressions of sarcasm or humorous abbreviations to describe the people in your care
- You should not falsify records
- Use black ink when writing records
- Do not use correction fluid in records

Thinking cap 16.3

Using abbreviations

Think about the abbreviations that you and your colleagues use in your day-to-day work. What is the purpose of using them? Can you think of any actual or potential problems associated with the use of abbreviations at work?

Making concerns known

You have a duty to make known any concerns you may have and report any unsafe or incompetent practice to your organisation or your organisation's regulatory body. If you consider that your manager has not taken your concerns seriously then you have a responsibility to make the report under the whistleblowing procedure. If the concerns that you have are about a person's information then you will have to seek their permission prior to making a complaint. If you have serious worries about the recording, storing or sharing of information, you should make a written record, noting your worries and to whom you have reported them. Sign, date and write your name on the record as this could be used as evidence at a later stage.

The use of social media

Social media and their use have become part of our everyday lives. Appropriate information exchange is key to the provision of safe and effective health and social care. The uses and types of electronic ways of communicating are growing, and this includes the use of social media. There are many advantages to using these various modes of communication, with the intention of improving care provision; there are also a number of potential drawbacks. When information has been made available publicly, for example on a website or through social media, it can be very difficult to remove or retrieve it. Information is shared instantaneously.

As a health or social care worker you should be careful to use social media responsibly, and at all times remember the confidentiality rights of all individuals, including the other people that you work with. Breaching confidentiality through use of social media, including the taking of or sharing of photos or videos, can result in the initiation of disciplinary procedures. In some cases this could even be a criminal offence depending on what is shared.

Apply common sense online, as you would in real life. The same standards of conduct that are expected of you in your daily professional practice are also relevant when using social media and electronic forms of communication. If you have a social media presence online, this should be kept separate from your professional identity.

Chapter summary

- As the use of information technology increases so too will the amount of personal information gathered and stored.
- There is a need for the secure handling of information in health and social care settings.
- Legislation relates to the recording, storage and sharing of information in health and social care.
- Specific aspects of the law are in place to ensure that information is handled in a safe, sensitive and legal manner.
- Failing to protect a person's personal information could result in that information being used inappropriately and illegally.
- There are eight principles associated with the Data Protection Act that will help to safeguard personal information.
- The Freedom of Information Act exists to provide public access to information held by public authorities.
- There are some aspects of information that might be withheld to protect various interests, and if this is the case, the person must be aware of it.
- Your organisation is legally obliged to put in place measures that will safeguard personal information regardless of whether the information is on a computer or is paper generated.
- With regards to the safe handling of information you should work in accordance with agreed ways of working.
- Your organisation should provide you with training on how to manage personal information.
- There are policies and procedures in place in your organisation concerning information and advice about handling information, how this is accessed and keeping information confidential. You should familiarise yourself with these policies and procedures.
- If you have any concerns over the recording, storing or sharing of information you should raise these with your colleagues or your manager and ensure that you record your concerns.
- If the information concerns the privacy of a person for whom you provide care or offer support then you must obtain consent from that person prior to passing the information on unless the information poses a risk to the person had it not been passed on.

- Ensure that you write your name, sign and date all records. All information recorded has to be legible and written in black ink and must be factual.
- Records, including care plans, have to be kept up to date and reviewed in accordance with local policy and procedure.
- You should be careful to use social media responsibly, taking into account the confidentiality rights of all individuals, including other people with whom you work.

Case scenario 16.1

Kelly-Ann

Kelly-Ann is a healthcare assistant who works in a GP surgery and she assists the practice nurse with a number of duties. Today she is taking part in new patient assessments. This requires Kelly-Ann to work with the patient in assessing their health and social care needs. A new patient, Darren, has just moved into the area and his notes have been transferred to the new surgery electronically. Kelly-Ann has this information on the screen.

The data on the screen contain much personal information about Darren. He has a history of being abused as a child and is receiving help and support from a psychologist concerning these traumatic events; Darren self-harms.

After the assessment has taken place, Kelly-Anne fails to log off from the system as the cleaner (Jasmine) tells her that she wants to come into the consultation room to clean it before the next patient arrives. Whilst cleaning the room Jasmine is able to see Darren's details on the screen and she realises that Darren is her daughter's boyfriend. Jasmine uses her smart phone to take photographs of the data on the screen.

In this scenario what measures should have been taken to reduce the risk of Darren's personal information being inappropriately accessed? If discovered how could Jasmine and Kelly-Ann be called to account for their actions and omission?

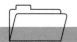

Resource file

GOV.UK
UK government website with information concerning the Data Protection Act.
https://www.gov.uk/data-protection/the-data-protection-act

Department of Health report on assistive technology
Assistive technology is any product or service designed to enable independence for disabled and older people.
https://www.gov.uk/government/uploads/system/uploads/attachment_data/file/211647/S22_Report_2012-13__2__FINAL.pdf

Health and Social Care Information Centre
Code of Practice on Confidential Information.
http://systems.hscic.gov.uk/infogov/codes/cop/code.pdf

Chapter 17

Infection prevention and control

Care certificate outcomes

1. Prevent the spread of infection.

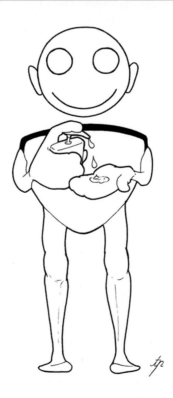

Fundamentals of Care: A Textbook for Health and Social Care Assistants, First Edition. Ian Peate.
© 2017 John Wiley & Sons Ltd. Published 2017 by John Wiley & Sons Ltd.

Take stock

Rate your current knowledge and skills prior to reading this chapter. Put a tick in the box that you think applies to you with regards to the standard being discussed:

Key:
I know this I have a good level of knowledge or skills regarding this aspect of the standard. I make use of the knowledge and skills identified on a regular basis, feeling confident in my ability and performance. I do not need a refresher.
Satisfactory My level of knowledge and standard of skills meet the criteria associated with the standard. I use the skills and knowledge from time to time. I might not always feel confident in my capability. I would benefit from a refresher.
I require a review I do not feel that I have the skills and/or the knowledge that would enable me to meet the standard in a confident and competent way. The knowledge and skills I used to have are no longer valid. I will require a refresher.
This is new to me I have never worked in a caring role before or I have never covered this topic before. I will need further training and development in this area.

Standard	Self-assessment			
Describe the modes of transmission	☐ I know this	☐ Satisfactory	☐ I should review this	☐ This is new to me
Outline the process of effective hand washing	☐ I know this	☐ Satisfactory	☐ I should review this	☐ This is new to me
Explain how inadequate health or hygiene may pose a risk to the people you support or provide care to	☐ I know this	☐ Satisfactory	☐ I should review this	☐ This is new to me
List the common types of personal protective clothing, equipment and procedures and how and when to use them	☐ I know this	☐ Satisfactory	☐ I should review this	☐ This is new to me
Explain the principles of safe handling of infected or soiled linen and clinical waste	☐ I know this	☐ Satisfactory	☐ I should review this	☐ This is new to me

Introduction

Infection prevention and control are essential components of health and social care. Infections cost millions of pounds per year to treat as well as causing people and their families unnecessary suffering and concern.

The steps taken to protect from infection those people that you care for or offer support to, as well as the other people you work with, represent an essential activity in the quality of care, particularly as there are some infections that have the ability to spread within environments where people who are susceptible share eating and living accommodation. It is also important to be aware of the possibility of infection and to identify any risks promptly.

Acquired infections can be serious and in some cases life threatening. These may make any underlying medical conditions worse and can negatively impact on a person's recovery. Some infections can be caused by organisms that are resistant to antibiotics. These types of infection have generated much media interest and this can cause alarm in the people you care for or offer support to as well as their relatives.

It is important that there is clear information on the standards of infection prevention and control where you work. The available information will allow you to make informed choices and enhance confidence in the quality of care and support offered. The people you care for and their families will want to be assured that the care and support their relatives and dependants are receiving is provided in a clean and safe environment.

Roles and responsibilities

It is the responsibility of employees to take precautionary measures to prevent and control the spread of infection in the workplace. This responsibility involves working safely to protect your-self, other members of staff, visitors and those you care for or offer support to from infections. Employers also have a responsibility to protect others, as laid down in law.

There are a number of obligations and duties placed on the employer. The employer is required to provide personal protective equipment (PPE), organise training for staff, undertake risk assessment, and ensure the general health and safety of staff in the work environment. It also has to ensure that those who use services are safe.

By informing all staff of infection prevention and control policies, procedures and updates can help to ensure that all staff are being provided with the necessary information to follow safe practices when working whilst adhering to the law. The employer also has a duty to ensure that staff are updated and attend training sessions when these are provided.

Stop, look, respond 17.1

Infection prevention and control updates

Locate where in your workplace the infection prevention and control policies are kept. Where would you find information should there be an infection outbreak?

You have a responsibility to keep up to date with your own vaccinations in line with the vaccination schedule. Being vaccinated can protect the people you care for or offer support to.

You should contact your manager before reporting for work if you have a cold or flu-like symptoms, an upset stomach or skin infections. If you have diarrhoea or vomiting then you should not go work until you have been symptom free for 48 hours.

As your clothes can become contaminated with harmful microorganisms, you are required to wear disposable aprons and oversleeves when handling anything contaminated with body fluids; these can help to protect your clothes from contamination. Change your clothes daily: this can reduce the possibility of any contaminants remaining on your clothing and being spread to the individuals you provide support for. If you wear a uniform or work clothing, this should be washed on a hot wash, tumble-dried or hot ironed with the intention of killing any bacteria present. At all times you should refer to agreed ways of working and local policy and procedure.

Daily washing, showering or bathing can remove most of the microorganisms on your skin. Personal hygiene is very important for those who take care of others. Your fingernails should be kept short. Apart from a plain wedding band, rings, wristwatches or bracelets must not be worn as these can make hand washing less effective. Any cuts should be covered with a waterproof dressing. Microorganisms can live on the skin and the number of pathogens increases when the skin has been damaged.

229

Transmission of infection

Infection prevention and control is required to prevent the transmission of communicable diseases in all health and social care settings. A basic understanding of infection prevention and control is required to identify, reduce and manage risks.

Healthcare-associated infections (HCAI) do not just affect people and staff in hospitals, HCAIs can occur in any healthcare setting, and these include general practice settings, clinics and dental surgeries as well as long-term care facilities. HCAIs are potentially preventable adverse happenings as opposed to an unpredictable complication. Anybody who works in or enters any healthcare facility is at risk of transmitting infection or being infected. When effective infection prevention and control procedures are implemented, this can significantly reduce the rate of infection.

Not all infections are preventable. However, managing infection control and ensuring best practice can significantly improve care outcomes and service user safety.

The human body plays host to microorganisms, most of which are welcome guests; however, some are infectious and can cause illness. In order to prevent and control the spread of infection you will need to understand how infections are spread or transmitted. The spreading of microbes is known as transmission, and the transmission of pathogens can occur in a number of ways.

When harmful germs, known as pathogens (or pathogenic microorganisms), enter the body and grow they can cause infection and infectious diseases. These microorganisms can only be seen by using a microscope as they are so small.

Unlike other diseases such as cancer, anaemia and asthma, infectious diseases can spread from one person to another person. Although cleanliness contributes to the control of infection, the prevention of infection demands more than just cleanliness. The health and social care worker has a key role to play in stopping the spread of pathogens – you can help to prevent and control infection.

Pathogens are organisms (individual living things) that can cause disease. They include microorganisms such as:

- bacteria;
- viruses;
- fungi;
- protozoa;
- parasites.

Table 17.1 provides a discussion of pathogenic organisms and some of the diseases that they may cause.

Some groups of people may be more susceptible or vulnerable to infection than others; for example:

Table 17.1 Pathogens and some diseases that they may cause

Pathogen	Discussion and disease
Bacteria	These have the ability to multiply very rapidly; at body temperature they can reach harmful levels very quickly. Meticillin-resistant *Staphylococcus aureus* (MRSA) is a harmful bacterium and so too is *Clostridium difficile* (*C. difficile*). Cholera is another example of a disease caused by a bacterium
Viruses	A virus can only multiply in living cells; they can survive on surfaces and also in food. Viruses can be transmitted (spread) from person to person and from the environment to food. It takes only a few viral organisms to cause illness Influenza is an illness caused by a virus; other examples include norovirus
Fungi	Most fungi are not dangerous, but some types are pathogenic and can be harmful to health. These organisms live on hosts Athlete's foot (tinea pedis), thrush (*Candida* infection) and ringworm (tinea) are caused by fungi
Protozoa	Pathogenic protozoa are parasitic single-celled organisms that can divide only within a host organism. Malaria is caused by a protozoan (*Plasmodium*)
Parasite	A parasite is an organism that lives in another organism (the host) and often harms it. It is dependent on its host for survival, and has to be in or on the host to live, grow and multiply. A parasite cannot live independently. Parasites are living things that use other living things – like the body – for food and a place to live. They can be transmitted through contaminated food or water, a bug bite, or sexual contact. Parasitic infections include bed bugs, body lice (pediculosis) and tapeworms

Table 17.2 Modes of transmission

Contact transmission	Droplet transmission	Airborne transmission
Contact transmission occurs when microorganisms are transferred as a result of direct physical contact between an infected person and a susceptible host Indirect transmission involves the passive transfer of an infectious agent to a susceptible host via an intermediate object or fomite (instruments, bed rails, bed tables and other environmental surfaces)	Occurs when respiratory droplets, i.e. produced by coughing, sneezing or talking, contact susceptible mucosal surfaces, e.g. eyes, nose or mouth. Can also occur indirectly via contact of hands with contaminated fomites and then mucosal surfaces. Respiratory droplets are large and unable to remain suspended in the air; they are frequently spread over short distances	Refers to infectious agents that are spread via droplet nuclei (residue from evaporated droplets) containing infective microorganisms. These organisms can live outside the body, staying suspended in the air for long periods, infecting others via upper and lower respiratory tracts

- Those who are very old or very young (the extremes of age).
- People who have problems with their immune system (e.g. people with cancer or those who have had an organ transplant).
- Those who are frail.
- The malnourished.
- People who live in conditions that lack good hygiene (the homeless).

When people who belong to these groups become infected then the symptoms they experience may be severe and serious and, in some instances this can be life threatening. It can be difficult to treat the infection if the microorganisms that cause the disease are resistant to antibiotics. Table 17.2 provides an overview of the modes of transmission.

The chain of infection

The path of transmission is known as the chain of infection. For an infection to develop each link in the chain must be connected (Figure 17.1). Breaking any of the links in the chain can stop the transmission of infection.

Infectious agent

The infectious agent is any microorganism that can cause a disease, for example a bacterium, virus, parasite, protozoan or fungus. Reasons that the organism will cause an infection are its ability to multiply and grow (virulence), the organism's ability to enter tissue (invasiveness) and its ability to cause disease (pathogenicity).

Reservoir

This is the place where the microorganism lives, flourishes and reproduces. The reservoir could be food, water, toys, sports equipment, door knobs, faeces or respiratory secretions.

Portal of exit

The portal of exit is the place where the organism leaves the reservoir, for example, open wounds, the respiratory tract (nose, mouth), intestinal tract (rectum), urinary tract (urethra) or blood and other body fluids.

Mode of transmission

This is the means by which an organism transfers from one carrier to another; this can be by either direct transmission (direct contact between an infectious host and a susceptible host) or indirect transmission (this involves an intermediate carrier such as an environmental surface or a piece of equipment).

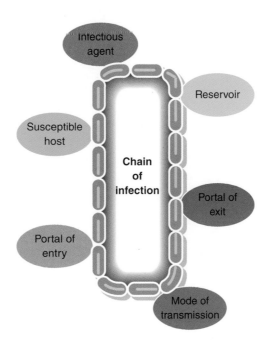

Figure 17.1 The chain of infection. *Source*: Peate I. (2016) *Medical-Surgical Nursing at a Glance*. Reproduced with permission of John Wiley & Sons Ltd.

Infectious diseases

The term 'Notification of infectious diseases' is used to refer to the legal duties for reporting notifiable diseases. In the list below identify those infectious diseases that have to be reported in accordance with the Health Protection (Notification) Regulations 2010.

Infection	Reportable Yes	Reportable No
Acute meningitis		
Botulism		
Cholera		
Diphtheria		
Food poisoning		
Glandular fever		
Hepatitis B		
Hepatitis C		
Herpes zoster		
HIV		
Influenza		
Legionnaires' disease		
Leprosy		
Malaria		
Measles		
Mumps		
Pneumonia		
Rabies		
Rosacea		
Rubella		
Syphilis		
Smallpox		
Tetany		
Tuberculosis		
Urinary tract infection		
Whooping cough		
Yellow fever		

Portal of entry

The portal of entry refers to the opening where an infectious disease enters the host's body. Examples include the mucous membranes, open wounds, urinary catheters or feeding tubes. Often this is the same as the portal of exit.

Susceptible host

The susceptible host is the person who is at risk for developing an infection. There are a number of factors that make a person more susceptible to disease, including defective immunisation, advanced age, underlying chronic disease (e.g. diabetes or asthma), conditions that damage the immune system, certain types of medication, the presence of invasive devices including feeding tubes and malnutrition.

Stop, look, respond 17.3

E. coli (Escherichia coli)

Write notes about one bacterium's journey – *E. coli* – and relate this to the chain of infection in the table below.

E. coli (*Escherichia coli*) is a bacterium. There are many strains (subtypes) of *E. coli*. Most strains live in the gut of healthy humans and animals. Usually they do not cause any harm and are one of the normal bacteria found in the gut. However, some strains of *E. coli* can cause various infections and diseases.

Aspect of the chain	Notes
The infectious agent is:	*E. coli*
Where can *E. coli* live and multiply (the reservoir)?	
To be transmitted onwards *E. coli* must find a portal of exit from the body; where is this?	
How can *E. coli* be transmitted; what is the mode of transmission?	
For infection with *E. coli* to occur the organism needs to find a means of entry to the body. What might the means of entry be?	
For infection to occur the person must be susceptible for the infection to take hold. What might make a person susceptible?	

Understanding the modes of transmission of infectious organisms and knowing how and when to apply the basic principles of infection prevention is key to controlling infection. This is the responsibility of everybody working in and visiting a healthcare facility.

Infectious agents are biological agents that cause disease or illness to their hosts. The most likely sources of infectious agents are the people being cared for or offered support and the health and social care workers, and these are also the most common susceptible hosts. The chain has to be broken to prevent onward transmission of infection.

Correct hand hygiene is the single most important activity for reducing the likelihood of infection and helping to control the spread of any illnesses. This is an important activity in all settings.

Breaking the chain

Many infections can be prevented. There are many opportunities for health and social care workers to break the chain of infection – stopping infection requires a break in the links of the chain. But some links are easier to break than others. Preventing a pathogen from entering a person is easier than stopping one from leaving an infected person.

The measures that are taken to protect from infection the people for whom you care or offer support, as well as other people you work with, are key measures of high-quality care and support. You have to work in ways that will prevent infection, because not everybody who has harmful microorganisms will be ill or demonstrate any symptoms. In every situation you must take standard precautions, which are the actions that should be taken to reduce the risk of infection (Table 17.3).

Effective hand hygiene

The single most important measure in preventing cross-infection is hand washing. The technique requires thorough cleaning, rinsing and drying of both hands. The principal route by which cross-infection occurs is the hands.

There have been a number of intensive efforts to implement stricter hand-washing policies in all health and social care settings; effective hand washing remains a key public health initiative. Hand washing is an essential aspect of any caregiver's range of skills. It is important to know what these skills are and how to carry them out in order to provide people with a safe environment.

Thinking cap 17.1

Effective hand washing

What do you think are the barriers to effective hand washing? How might these be overcome?

Hand washing is an automatic behaviour that is undertaken by all in homes, schools and other environments. The overall aim of effective hand washing is to prevent the transmission of microorganisms between people or between other living things and people. Inanimate objects and surfaces, for example contaminated cutlery or clinical equipment, can put the health and wellbeing of a person at risk.

Using the correct technique in order to wash hands can not only save lives but also save money (Figure 17.2). Poor hand-washing practices can lead to urinary tract infections, blood-stream infections, respiratory infections and infection of wounds. These infections are caused by the transfer of microorganisms from staff and families to vulnerable people; using the correct hand-washing procedures could prevent these.

Table 17.3   Standard precautions

- Effective hand hygiene
- Safe disposal of waste
- Safe management of laundry
- Correct use of personal protective equipment (PPE)

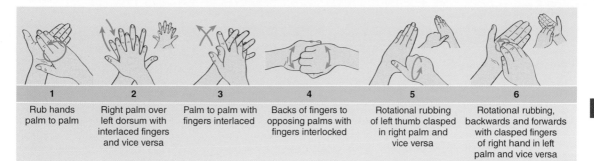

1	2	3	4	5	6
Rub hands palm to palm	Right palm over left dorsum with interlaced fingers and vice versa	Palm to palm with fingers interlaced	Backs of fingers to opposing palms with fingers interlocked	Rotational rubbing of left thumb clasped in right palm and vice versa	Rotational rubbing, backwards and forwards with clasped fingers of right hand in left palm and vice versa

Figure 17.2   Hand-washing technique. *Source*: Reproduced with permission of WHO.

In all environments hand washing is compulsory and this must be carried out using recognised policies and procedures. There are several practices associated with hand hygiene, such as using alcohol hand rubs and the act of physically washing the hands. When the correct procedures are not used there are a number of consequences, including the devastating impact this can have on the health and wellbeing of the person you are caring for or offering support to.

Hands must be decontaminated before you make direct contact with the people being cared for or supported, and after any activity or contact that contaminates the hands, including when gloves are removed. Alcohol hand gels and rubs are a practical alternative to soap and water; however, alcohol is not a cleaning agent. Hands that are visibly dirty or potentially grossly contaminated must be washed with soap and water and dried thoroughly. Whenever feasible, staff should have access to the means to clean their hands at the point of care, and where possible soap and water should be used. However, this is not always possible with the placement of sinks.

Detergent wipes should be used if soap and water are not available, and this should be followed by drying the hands thoroughly with paper towels or air drying, then alcohol gel can be used. Only use alcohol gel if the hands are visibly clean; using alcohol gel on contaminated hands renders the solution ineffective. Detergent wipes and hand rubs should be readily available at the point of care. Alcohol gel should be used between performing different care activities with the same patient. See Figure 17.3 for the five moments of hand washing.

Safe disposal of waste

The place where you work will have a waste handling policy outlining how you should manage different types of waste. At all times you have to ensure that you understand and follow this policy.

There are different requirements for how waste should be handled safely to protect yourself, those you work with and the people whom you provide care and support for. Clinical waste is placed in either yellow or orange plastic sacks; it should be kept separate from other types of waste and has to be disposed of using specialist facilities. Clinical waste may be either hazardous (waste that poses or may pose a risk of infection, such as pads and dressings) or non-hazardous (this is non-infectious waste). Waste containers should be handled carefully to avoid contamination. You should not use your hands to open the lids of bins; these should be pedal-type bins. PPE should be used to protect yourself from contamination and infection where appropriate.

Thinking cap 17.2

Waste management

How is waste managed in the place where you work? What do the various coloured bags mean and what types of waste should they be used for?

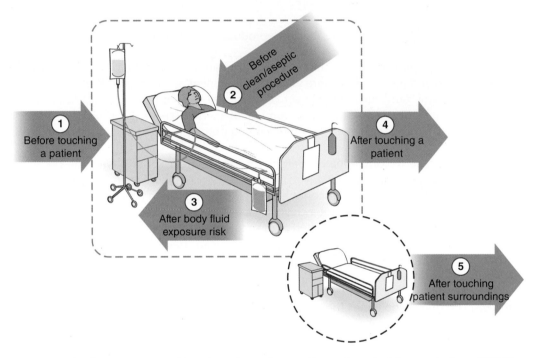

Figure 17.3   The five moments of hand washing. *Source*: Reproduced with permission of WHO.

Sharps disposal

An essential aspect of infection prevention and control is the safe handling and disposal of sharps. There are a number of sharps bins available depending on the environment and reason for disposal. Sharps include needles, scalpels, stitch cutters, glass ampoules, bone fragments and any sharp instrument. The main hazards of a sharps injury are bloodborne viruses, such as hepatitis B, hepatitis C and HIV. Unsafe or poor practice can result in injury to yourself or others; for example, cleaners may experience injuries as a result of sharps being misplaced in waste bins. Sharps injuries are preventable, and learning following incidents helps to prevent repeat accidents. To reduce the risk of injury and exposure to bloodborne viruses, it is essential that sharps are used safely and disposed of carefully:

- Sharps must be disposed of at the point of use into an approved container.
- A sharps bin should bear the name of the person who assembled it and the date of assembly on the label. This also applies to the individual closing the bin.

- Sharps bins should not be filled past the 'full' line marked on the bin.
- Bins should always be kept above floor level and out of reach of children to prevent unauthorised access.
- If transporting sharps by car, these should be kept in the boot of the car.
- Never pass sharps from one hand to the other.
- Do not handle sharps more than is essential.
- Never replace protective covering (resheath) on needles.
- Do not bend or break needles.
- Never separate a needle from its syringe before disposing of them.

Thinking cap 17.3

Sharps

In the area where you work how would you dispose safely of sharps? What types of sharps are in your workplace?

Safe management of laundry

The provision of clean linen and clothing is a fundamental aspect of care. The incorrect handling and storage of linen can pose an infection hazard. Organisations have a variety of different laundry systems and equipment. Therefore it is important to understand what system is being used where you work and why.

Soiled linen must be managed in accordance with local policy and agreed ways of working. Linen coming into contact with workers or others can become contaminated as a result of harmful microorganisms and body fluids. Personal protective equipment must be worn when handling linen that is infected as this has the potential to transfer pathogens to skin and clothing. All infected linen (linen that is contaminated with body fluids) must be washed separately from other items.

- Items should only be washed in a dedicated laundry room using the correct process. Clothing can be decontaminated in a 40–50°C wash followed by tumble-drying or hot ironing.
- Bedding and towels should be washed in a hot wash to ensure that bacteria are killed.
- Used linen and clothing must always be kept in laundry bags or baskets and not loose on the floor.
- Laundry should be moved to the washing area in sealed, colour-coded bags.
- When supporting an individual in their own home you should seek permission to wash infected linen.
- When handling laundry you should always wear gloves and an apron and carry out hand hygiene.
- Clean linen should be stored in a dry area above floor level and must not be stored with used linen.

Thinking cap 17.4

Laundry and linen

Are there any specific policies and procedures in place where you work that inform you and your colleagues of how to manage linen? Where are they located? Who would you go to for advice?

Personal protective equipment (PPE)

Personal protective equipment (PPE) is used to protect health and social care workers and others from risk of infection; it is essential for health and safety. The selection of PPE is based on an assessment of the risk of transmission of microorganisms to the person being cared for or to the health or social care worker, and the risk of contamination of the health or social care worker's clothing and skin/mucous membranes by the person's blood, body fluids, secretions and excretions.

The risk of infection is reduced by preventing the transmission of microorganisms to the person via the hands of staff or vice versa. Gloves are also required for contact with hazardous chemicals and some pharmaceuticals, such as disinfectants or cytotoxic drugs. PPE includes items such as gloves, aprons, masks, goggles or visors.

Stop, look, respond 17.4

Personal protective equipment

There are instances when as part of your work you are required to use PPE. Your employer provides you with the appropriate materials and equipment to protect you from possible injury and from the risk of infection while you are at work. In the table below list five examples of common types of personal protective clothing, equipment and procedures and how and when you might use them.

Types of personal protective clothing, equipment and procedures	How and when you would have to use it

Chapter summary

- Infection prevention and control are crucial elements of health and social care.
- Infections cost millions of pounds per year to treat. They also cause unnecessary suffering and concern to the people affected and their families.
- There are several ways in which infection can enter the body. Understanding these will help ensure that you and the people you provide care and support to are safe and that the risk of infection is reduced.
- Infectious diseases can be transmitted from person to person.
- Working according to local policy and adhering to procedure can help to stop the spread of pathogens and prevent and control infection.
- Most pathogens that enter the body and grow are microorganisms, so small they can be seen only through a microscope.

- Pathogenic organisms include bacteria, viruses, fungi, protozoa and parasites.
- The chain of infection is made up of six different links: pathogen, reservoir, portal of exit, means of transmission, portal of entry and susceptible host.
- Each link has a unique role in the chain. In order for the spread of infectious diseases to occur the chain of infection must be completed.
- Preventing infection means interrupting or breaking the links in the chain so as to prevent the transmission of infection.
- There are several actions that can be taken to break the chain of infection.
- Each health and social care worker has a key role to play in preventing infection. You must ensure you are aware of and use local policy and procedure.
- It is your responsibility to keep up to date with your own vaccinations. You should speak to your manager before coming to work if you are ill.
- Your manager has a duty to provide you with personal protective equipment that you need to protect you from injury and, as far as possible, from the risk of infection while you are at work.
- Effective hand washing is one activity that can reduce transmission risk.
- It is important you understand how different types of waste should be handled safely.
- You and your employer are responsible for reducing risk of injury with regards to the management and safe disposal of sharps.
- There are agreed ways of working concerning linen. All infected linen must be managed in specific ways and must be washed separately from other items.

Case scenario 17.1

Ulli and Bayla

Ulli works as a healthcare assistant in a residential care home. She has been working there for the last three weeks. She is currently working on the night shift.

One of the residents, Bayla, has become increasingly unwell throughout the day. The day staff say she seems to be confused and is complaining of abdominal pain, she has a temperature, she appears flushed and she has been incontinent of urine, which is unlike her; her urine appears dark and is malodorous.

The night staff are concerned that she is getting worse and they have made the decision to call her GP; they have informed Bayla of this. The GP night service doctor arrives and with the assistance of Ulli, who is also acting as Bayla's chaperone, the GP examines Bayla; amongst other things he takes blood from Bayla for analysis.

The GP has left and Ulli is clearing away after his visit. Ulli attempts to resheath the used needle that the GP has left and in doing so she sustains a needle-stick injury when clearing up the used needle and syringe from Bayla's bedside table.

What steps should Ulli and her manager now take after Ulli reports that she has injured herself with Bayla's used needle?

How can needle-stick injuries and sharps injuries be prevented?

Resource file

Infection Prevention Society
The Infection Prevention Society aspires to lead, shape and inform the infection prevention agenda locally, nationally and internationally.
http://www.ips.uk.net

NHS Employers. Prevention of sharps injuries
The voice of employers in the NHS, supporting them to put patients first.
http://www.nhsemployers.org/your-workforce/retain-and-improve/staff-experience/health-work-and-wellbeing/protecting-staff-and-preventing-ill-health/partnership-working-across-your-organisation/health--safety/new-eu-regulations-to-protect-healthcare-workers-from-sharps-injuries

RCN Infection Prevention and Control Network
This UK and international network is for those who have an interest in infection prevention, regardless of practice setting or role.
https://www.rcn.org.uk/get-involved/forums/infection-prevention-and-control-network

Introduction

There may be occasions when you will have questions or queries that you want answers to and you might want help with finding answers. This chapter will consider a range of issues that you might encounter as you strive to provide high-quality, safe and effective care.

Asking questions and seeking support or guidance should never be seen as a weakness and you should never shy away from this. You should make known any concerns or issues that you face in the workplace. The chapter does not provide answers to the questions raised; it merely encourages you to think around the issues and apply your knowledge in helping to arrive at an answer.

I am asked to carry out an activity that I have not done before and my supervisor insists that I do it. She says the others do it so why don't I? What should I do?

When you provide care to or offer support to other people you must have their best interests at the forefront of your mind. Your key aim is to provide people with safe and effective care; doing something to or with somebody that you have not been deemed competent to do could cause harm to the person you are caring for.

The Code of Conduct for Healthcare Support Workers and Adult Social Care Workers in England notes that you should be honest with yourself and others about what you can do. You need to be able to recognise your abilities as well as the limitations of your competence, and you must only carry out those tasks that have been agreed in your job description (sometimes referred to as agreed ways of working) and for which you are competent.

Speak with your supervisor and explain why you will not carry out the procedure. Spend time explaining that you do not feel competent, that you need some more training, an update or extra supervision. Saying no for the right reason – to ensure that the person you are caring for or offer support to is safe – is the right thing to do.

You must tell your supervisor or employer about any issues that you think might affect your ability to do your job in a competent and safe manner. If you do not feel competent to carry out an activity, you must report this. Acting in this way enables you to recognise both the extent and the limits of your role.

You should remember that competence is associated with the knowledge, skills, attitudes and ability to carry out your work safely and effectively without the need for direct supervision, and being competent requires you to possess the necessary ability, knowledge, or skill to do something in a successful way.

My line manager (a registered nurse) often leaves me in charge whilst he leaves the care home at night and I am not sure this is a good thing. Should I be doing something about this?

The issues of accountability and delegation are important ones that all staff should take seriously, and this also includes your manager. The values and principles that are associated with accountability and delegation apply to all members of the team, including healthcare assistants, advanced practitioners, registered nurses, and other registered practitioners as well as nursing students.

Many different people, all with different skills, knowledge and competence, contribute to the care of people who live in care homes. Each member of staff can make a positive or negative

Questions you always wanted to ask

Care certificate outcomes

There are no care certificate outcomes for this chapter. This chapter aims to:

- Provide guidance on a range of issues that may arise in the health or care setting.
- Support the health and care worker in addressing questions, queries and concerns that they may have or have experienced in the workplace.

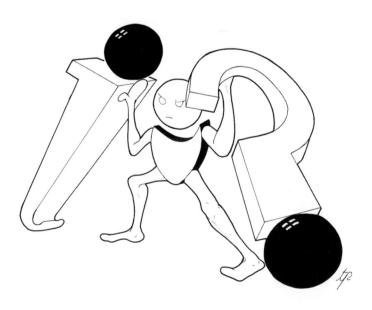

Fundamentals of Care: A Textbook for Health and Social Care Assistants, First Edition. Ian Peate.
© 2017 John Wiley & Sons Ltd. Published 2017 by John Wiley & Sons Ltd.

contribution to the resident's care experience. The person in charge of a patient's nursing care is usually a registered nurse. There are times, however, when the registered nurse may need to delegate some tasks as nurses cannot perform every intervention or activity for every patient.

Prior to any activity being delegated to you, adequate instructions should be provided as well as ensuring that you are able to do the work competently. If unclear about the appropriateness of the delegation, you should seek advice and assistance from those more experienced than yourself.

One of the most complex and sometimes difficult skills any manager working in the fields of health and social care must master is that of delegation. It requires sophisticated clinical judgment and final accountability for patient care. Effective delegation is based on an understanding of the concepts of responsibility, authority and accountability. Inappropriate delegation can result in negative health and wellbeing outcomes. When there is ineffective delegation, the quality of care can be diminished and valuable resources can be mismanaged. Being clear about what can be delegated helps to define high-quality professional practice for those who offer care and support to others, for other team members, patients and their families.

The employer needs to ensure that you have been assessed as competent to carry out the duties that are required of you; this is about ability. Being required to be in charge whilst the line manager leaves the premises has to be part of your job description and this is associated with your responsibility. The line manager who has delegated this activity is deemed to have the authority to do this but only in full knowledge of competences and the job description. At all times the line manager retains the professional responsibility of appropriate delegation and although not currently regulated you too are accountable for your actions.

If a manager has delegated duties to a health or social care worker and he or she believes they do not have the required competency, or that it is an inappropriate delegation, then he or she should refuse the instruction. This must then be raised formally in writing with the employer.

A lady I care for has asked me to act as a witness to her last will and testament. She wants me to sign a form as she has no other family. Should I do this? It is only my signature after all.

There is nothing to prevent a health or care support worker from acting as a witness to a will. However you would be strongly advised against doing this, as you have a close connection with the person. A person who is completely independent or who does not have any interest in the person's care would be a more appropriate person to witness this. There may be policies and procedures in use in your workplace that would guide you with regards to this.

Those people who express a wish to make a will, and who are capable of managing their own affairs, should be advised to consult their own solicitor or provision should be made for the solicitor to visit them. Consideration should also be given as to whether pastoral support (with the person's permission) for the person is appropriate; this can be obtained from hospital chaplains or other community faith groups.

It must be acknowledged that helping people and their families who wish to make a will, particularly in emotional and stressful circumstances, is an important activity. There are certain actions that need to be taken to ensure that any will is both lawful and valid. To be valid a will must be in writing (including typewriting) and has to be signed by the person in the presence of two witnesses who both sign their signatures in the presence of each other. Both witnesses must be present during the whole time that the person is signing their name. The witness is only witnessing the person's signature not the content of the will itself.

The health and support worker must treat as confidential the fact that the person they are caring for or offering support to has made a will unless the person consents to the disclosure of this fact to family or friends. Any request by a patient to make a will and the measures instituted, particularly where any doubt exists as to the patient's capacity, should be documented clearly in the person's notes or medical records.

A resident with a learning disability tells me that another resident is threatening him and taunting him because of his weight. What should I do about this?

An acceptance of abuse or bullying from whatever source will eventually, if permitted to continue, lead to a culture that is damaging. There should be a zero tolerance of abuse whoever it is perpetrated by.

The place where you work may have policy and procedures, for example on anti-bullying, managing distress or challenging behaviours, and safeguarding adults, and you should have undertaken appropriate training. The policy would cover abuse of a service user by another service user.

Your key aim is to take action that can support and protect both the victim and the alleged perpetrator and prevent abuse of this nature happening in the future. Abuse of one adult by another adult must be reported through the safeguarding adults procedure in the same way that other concerns of abuse and neglect would be reported. An assessment of risk of harm must be undertaken by a person who is competent to do so and appropriate actions taken thereafter.

If you are worried that there is an immediate danger of harm to a person then you should contact the police. If you think the person is in immediate risk of serious harm from physical violence then you should dial 999 for the emergency services.

Safeguarding adults is concerned with protecting those at risk of harm (vulnerable adults) from suffering abuse or neglect. Abuse can happen anywhere – at home, in a residential or nursing home, in a hospital, at work or in the street. There are different types of abuse, including emotional abuse or bullying, being humiliated or put down, or made to feel anxious or frightened.

Often, people who need safeguarding help are elderly and frail, living alone at home, or without much family support in care homes. Others at risk of suffering harm are those with physical or learning disabilities or people with mental health needs.

You can seek help by talking to, for example, your co-workers, your manager, a GP or doctor, a social worker or care manager, community or district nurses, daycare workers or hospital staff.

I am worried about a co-worker. She is very forgetful and often she arrives late for work looking very tired and there are times when I can smell alcohol on her breath. Should I report her?

The safety of the people to whom you offer care or support is paramount; you must take all steps to ensure they are safe and you must be vigilant in your actions. Any concerns you have that a person's health and wellbeing might be jeopardised must be reported. It is acknowledged that this may not be an easy situation to be in. But if you fail to report your concerns you could be jeopardising the care, health and safety of others including your co-worker.

What you are not required to do is to prejudge a person based on your subjective thoughts. Your workplace may have processes in place that will help you to ensure that you are not being discriminatory in any way but, at the same time, you are doing your duty to protect others. The policy may state to whom you must make known your concerns, and you should do this by providing factual information, not hearsay or conjecture. A possible outcome of your action may be that the person concerned receives help and support, and this might make a positive difference to the life of that member of staff.

I have been asked to write a witness statement concerning an untoward incident that occurred when I was on duty. Is this something I should do and if so how do I do this?

There are a number of reasons why healthcare or support workers may be required to write a witness statement and for some this can be a scary experience. It is not unusual for a person to be anxious or worried about writing a statement.

A witness statement is a written account of an event or happening that has occurred. The witness statement aims to provide information during an investigation or a disciplinary hearing. The witness statement, it should be remembered, is a legal document and as such this can be used as evidence during these and other hearings. When writing a witness statement you must therefore always provide a truthful and accurate account of the event.

There are many reasons why a statement is required to be written, such as:

- If a complaint has been made by a person who is being or has been given care or support. Such complaints are always investigated, and as part of this process, you and others who may have been involved in that person's care may be required to write a statement. There are policies in place for managing complaints.
- If a person has hurt themselves, their condition has seriously deteriorated or if something unpredicted has happened. Sometimes these are known as Serious Untoward Incidents, and those involved in the person's care may be asked to write a statement.
- If there is an investigation concerning you or other members of staff, for example if you or others with whom you work have a grievance or if an investigation proceeds to a disciplinary hearing; these are reasons why your employer might ask for a statement to be written.
- If there is a legal case, for example a statement for a coroner's report or court case.

Your organisation may have a format or template for statement writing, and if this is the case this should be used. If you have been asked to write a statement always seek advice from your trade union representative regardless of why you are being asked to provide the statement. Be sure, prior to submission, that they read it for you.

A witness statement is a legal document and it has to be legible and easy for anyone to read. Ensure that you always keep copies of your statements and store them in a safe place. Provide your trade union representative with a copy of your written statement. You are required always to provide a truthful and accurate account of the event that has taken place.

The statement should relate factual information and therefore should be about what you saw, what you know took place. It is never about what another person has told you happened or what they saw. You should never make assumptions; remember it is about fact.

If you have been asked to write a statement about someone who has been in your care or someone you have offered support to, you can ask to see the notes or documents so as to remind you of any involvement that you had. When writing a statement, however, you have to distinguish between the facts that have been written in the notes and documents and what you recall.

Take your time to write your statement, remember this is a legal document. An employer may tell you that they need it within a specific period of time; whilst it may help them to have it within this time, this is your statement and you should take time to ensure that you are happy with the content and accuracy. No one should change your statement without your permission.

Remember:

- Be completely honest and state if you cannot remember something.
- Avoid ambiguity or subjective statements.
- Avoid opinion or speculation; state facts only.
- Avoid abbreviations or jargon.
- Explain, if appropriate, why you made the decisions you did or took a particular form of action.
- Retain a copy for yourself.
- Seek advice from your trade union before submitting your statement.

I work in a residential home and I am petrified that one of the residents will die whilst I am on duty. How should I cope with this? I know it sounds daft but it really worries me.

The anxiety experienced demonstrates total commitment, honesty and dedication. Those involved in caring for people who are dying or have a terminal illness are faced with the process of dying; indeed, you are required to develop a meaningful relationship with the people you care for or offer support to. Working with these people and their families can be emotionally demanding and challenging, and most people working in a healthcare setting will encounter people who are at the end of their life. We each have our own personal attitude and response to death, and each healthcare worker's individual viewpoint can impact on the person who is dying. Providing good care or offering support to others at the end of their life requires an internal commitment on your part and this can take its toll.

It is totally understandable that you may have concerns about this very emotive issue – most people do. Those who provide care or offer support to others are human, and death and dying will have an impact on these people just as they impact on the people being cared for and their families.

There is no set approach to managing and coping with your first death. This is dependent on a number of things: for example, the type of death – was it peaceful and expected, or was it unexpected or traumatic? There are many textbooks available on coping with death and dying that may help to prepare you.

Often talking with co-workers and reflecting on events is a helpful coping strategy in getting through your first death. But nobody else knows what you are going through. If you do not talk about things, if you bottle things up, this may have implications for how you cope (or do not cope) in the future. Managers may provide you with time to speak about your fears and anxieties and they may encourage you to talk individually or with others. Some organisations hold voluntary debriefings after a death has occurred. What is required is that you feel safe to grieve and talk about what is on your mind.

Many feelings have been described with regards to death and dying, such as sadness, vulnerability, helplessness and empathy when interacting with dying individuals and their families. Offering people support or caring for them as they die can also provide feelings of satisfaction in so far as the person has had a peaceful death with dignity and compassion. Some regard this as a privilege, to be with the person and their family at this time, an honour and very special.

I am a lone worker and there are times when I am out and about and I feel scared and threatened. I have asked for a panic alarm to carry with me but my boss says I am just being silly. Should I just get on with it?

Your health and safety are of paramount importance. You should seek support and advice from others such as your trade union, letting them know of your fears and anxieties concerning lone working.

It is not illegal to work alone and in most cases it is perfectly safe to do so (e.g. a support worker employed to work in a person's home). The law requires, however, that employers ensure that their employees are 'reasonably' safe whilst working alone. The employer is required to consider the health and safety risks of the job being undertaken as well as any risks that may be caused by the employee working alone. If a risk assessment demonstrates that work cannot be carried out safely by a lone worker then arrangements for providing help or back up must be put in place. These measures should be implemented promptly.

There are some employees who may need special adjustments to manage any additional risk and these include:

- pregnant workers;
- young workers (those under 18 years of age);
- disabled workers;
- female workers (in some roles) (it must be noted that being a woman in itself is not a special condition).

Employers have to check that their employees have no medical conditions that will make them unsuitable for working alone. If this is the case they may need to seek medical advice in certain cases. If working conditions are reasonable and you are unable to carry out the job due to a medical condition, consideration will need to be given to another role; the employer only needs to make reasonable adaptations.

If a member of staff is working alone away from base, there should be procedures for leaving details of their work schedule for the day, their expected arrival and departure times, contact names and telephone numbers. There should be a system for lone workers to keep in contact and for raising the alarm if necessary.

New technology may provide ways of keeping in contact, and the manager should consider this. However, consideration should be given to its limitations and the circumstances in which it would be used. Personal alarms can be made available to staff and this may be as the result of a risk assessment.

It should be remembered that lone worker devices such as a personal alarm will not prevent incidents from occurring. They will not make people invincible and they should not be used in such a way that could be seen to intimidate, harass or coerce someone. If used correctly along with robust procedures, they will enhance the protection of lone workers. Lone workers should always exercise caution even if equipped with such devices and continue to use the dynamic risk assessment process. If a device is issued it will only be useful if checked regularly, properly maintained and kept fully charged.

I want to train to become a social worker but I don't have the required qualifications that the university is asking for. Are there other options open to me?

The entry criteria required to undertake training as a social worker, or for any other healthcare profession, for example a nurse, occupational therapist or physiotherapist, are set by the university that offers these programmes of study. There is a range of other requirements apart from academic qualifications that also need to be met, such as passing a range of tests (maths and English) and attending for interview.

Some universities may accept equivalents to the advertised criteria and they may take your experience as a health or support worker into account. You should contact the university and if possible arrange to speak with the admissions tutor, who may be able to guide you.

Your local college of further education may also be able to offer you advice about study opportunities that can help you achieve your career ambitions.

A person I provided care and support to has asked me out on a date. I used to know him when he worked in the same company I worked for, and he had an accident at work. Am I allowed to go on a date with him?

Those who provide healthcare and offer support to those who are unable to care or support themselves are very often respected and trusted by society. This reflects the special relationship and bond that those who care for others (often those who are vulnerable or at a vulnerable point in their lives) have with the recipients of that care. People expect the health or social care worker to act in their best interests and to respect their dignity. This means the person caring for or offering support to others should abstain from personal gain and from jeopardising the unique therapeutic relationship. You should be knowledgeable about professional boundaries and rules that govern these, which may be laid down in your contract of employment or in your Code of Conduct.

A therapeutic relationship is one that permits those who care for others to apply their professional knowledge, skills, abilities and experiences towards meeting the health and social care needs of the person. This unique and privileged relationship is dynamic, goal-oriented and patient-centred as it is designed to meet the person's needs. Regardless of the context or length of interaction, the therapeutic relationship protects the person's dignity, autonomy and privacy, allowing for the development of trust and respect.

Professional boundaries are those spaces between the power of the health and social care worker and the person's vulnerability. The power arises from the member of staff's position and their access to sensitive personal information. What the care worker knows about the individual's personal information greatly outweighs what the person knows about the care worker, and this results in an imbalance in the relationship. Every effort should be made to respect the power imbalance and ensure a person-centred relationship.

If a health or social care worker wants to date or even marry a former patient, then this must be given careful consideration by all parties. The following are important factors to consider when making this determination:

- What time has elapsed between the ending of their professional relationship and the start of their personal relationship?

- What kind of therapy did the person receive? Assisting a person with a short-term problem, such as a broken limb, is different than providing long-term care for a chronic condition or those who may have a mental health problem.
- What is the nature of the knowledge the health or social care worker has had access to and how will that affect the future relationship?
- Will the person need further therapy in the future?
- Is there risk to the person?

Chapter summary

- Throughout your career there will be many occasions when you will be seeking answers to questions that can impact on your own health and the health and wellbeing of others.
- Asking questions and seeking support or guidance is not a weakness and you should never shy away from this. You should always make known any concerns or issues that you face in the workplace.
- You should always adhere to local policy and procedure as you undertake your work.
- You should never undertake any activity or provide any element of care that you have not been deemed competent for as you could cause harm to the person you are caring for, yourself and also other others you work with.
- Before you accept any delegated activity you should be provided with adequate instructions and be deemed competent to undertake the task. If you are unclear about the appropriateness of the delegation, seek advice and assistance from those more experienced than yourself.
- It should be documented clearly in the person's notes or medical records if a person has requested to make a will and the measures instituted, particularly where any doubt exists as to the patient's capacity.
- An acceptance of abuse or bullying will eventually, if permitted to continue, lead to a culture that is damaging. There should be a zero tolerance of abuse whoever it is perpetrated by.
- The safety of the people to whom you offer care or support is paramount. You may be required to report any concerns you have that a person's health and wellbeing are in jeopardy.
- There are several reasons why healthcare or support workers may be asked to write a witness statement, and for some this can be an intimidating experience. It is not unusual for a person to be scared or worried about writing a statement.
- Providing good care or offering support to others at the end of their life requires an internal commitment on your part and this can take its toll.
- As a lone worker your health and safety are of paramount importance. Seek support and advice from others, such as your trade union, letting them know of your fears and anxieties in relation to lone working.
- If you are considering furthering your career, for example by studying at a university, there are some universities that might accept equivalents to the advertised criteria, taking your experience as a health or support worker into account. Contact the university and arrange to speak with the admissions tutor, who may be able to guide you.
- You should be knowledgeable about professional boundaries and any rules that govern these, which may be laid down in the contract of employment or in a Code of Conduct.

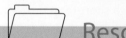

Resource file

UNISON

This is a trade union representing full-time and part-time staff who provide public services. They provide a range of advice regarding a variety of work-related issues.
www.unison.org.uk

Royal College of Nursing

A trade union and professional organisation representing nurses and healthcare assistants (the extended nursing family). The organisation provides work-related and professional advice.
www.rcn.org.uk

Universities and Colleges Admissions Service (UCAS)

This organisation's key role is to operate the admissions process for British universities. Services provided by UCAS include several online application portals, a number of search tools, and free information and advice directed at various audiences, including students considering higher education.
www.ucas.com

Health and Care Professions Council (HCPC)

A health and care professions regulator set up to protect the public. It maintains a register of health and care professionals who meet HCPC standards for training, professional skills, behaviour and health.
www.hcpc-uk.org

Nursing and Midwifery Council (NMC)

This organisation regulates nurses and midwives in England, Wales, Scotland and Northern Ireland. It exists to protect the public, setting standards of education, training, conduct and performance, so that nurses and midwives can deliver high-quality healthcare throughout their careers.
www.nmc.org.uk

Annotated bibliography

Chapter 1

King's Fund (2014) *Managing Quality in Community Health Care*. King's Fund, London.
Community healthcare services provide vital care out of hospital for millions of people. These range from children's services to care for older people and end-of-life support. The community sector plays a key part in meeting the challenges facing the health and care system. This report presents findings from a small-scale study into how quality is managed in community services, exploring how community care providers define and measure quality.

National Health Service (2014) *Understanding the New NHS*. NHS England, London.
Provides an overview of the new NHS, and explains the changes that have been made to the NHS. This applies to England.

Wild, K. (2014) Nursing: past, present and future. In: Peate, I., Nair, M. and Wild, K. (eds) *Nursing Knowledge and Practice*. John Wiley & Sons, Ltd, Oxford: Chapter 1, pp. 2–14.
This chapter provides insight into various aspects of health and social care and considers issues from the past, present and future.

Chapter 2

Ellis, P. and Bach, S. (2015) *Leadership Management and Team Working in Nursing*, 2nd edn. Learning Matters, Exeter.
Covers all of the core theory and knowledge, encouraging the reader to explore their own values and experiences when it comes to leadership. This will help to develop emotional intelligence and a solid understanding of what good leadership and management practice look like and why it matters to them.

Royal College of Nursing (2013) *We Think you are Amazing: HCAs and APs Valued Members of the Nursing Team*. RCN, London.
Highlights the role and function of the healthcare assistant and assistant practitioner. Provides discussion concerning the contribution healthcare support workers make.

Sanderson, H. and Lepkowsky, M.B. (2014) *Person-Centred Teams: A Practical Guide to Delivering Personalisation Through Effective Team-work*. Jessica Kingsley Publishers, London.
Practice Development Workbook for Nursing, Health and Social Care Teams provides a wide-ranging selection of activities, tools and resources covering vital aspects of practice development.

Chapter 3

Rawles, Z. (2014) *Essential Knowledge and Skills for Healthcare Assistants*. CRC Press, Boca Raton, FL.
Discusses the knowledge required to provide the safest and most effective patient care possible. Offers comprehensive coverage of both primary and secondary care settings with an emphasis on the role in primary care.

Royal College of Nursing (2015) *Accountability and Delegation. A Guide for the Nursing Team*. RCN, London.
This publication emphasises the fact that the nursing team is made up of many different people bringing with them a range of skills, knowledge and competence. It discusses the principles of accountability and delegation that can be applied to various staff and settings.

Welsh Assembly Government (2011) *Code of Conduct for Health and Social Care Workers in Wales*. Welsh Assembly Government, Cardiff.
The Code of Conduct sets the standard of conduct expected of health and social care workers. It outlines the behaviour and attitudes that you should expect from those workers signed up to the Code. It helps them to provide safe, compassionate care and support. This Code applies to Wales; other UK countries also have Codes of Conduct.

Chapter 4

Alsop, A. (2013) *Continuing Professional Development in Health and Social Care: Strategies for Lifelong Learning*. John Wiley & Sons, Ltd, Oxford.
Reflects the CPD requirements, reviews current policy on CPD, and discusses the theoretical basis for maintaining competence and for adult learning, whilst providing practical guidance on how to develop a strategy for professional and career development.

Innes, J. (2012) *The CV Book: Your Definitive Guide to Writing the Perfect CV*, 2nd edn. Pearson, Harlow.
Provides helpful hints and tips with regards to CV writing. The book supports the first-time and experienced CV writer.

Royal College of Nursing (2011) *Step by Step: Personal and Professional Development Opportunities for Health Care Assistants and Assistant Practitioners*. RCN, London.
Offers an overview of the various roles and functions that can be undertaken as a healthcare assistant and assistant practitioner. Concentrates on learning and development needs.

Chapter 5

Care Quality Commission (2015) *Regulation 20: Duty of Candour: Information for all Providers – NHS Bodies, Adult Social Care, Primary Medical and Dental Care, and Independent Healthcare*. CQC, Newcastle.
Discusses the Duty of Candour, a new CQC regulation that is applicable to all providers. The duty of candour is based on openness, transparency and candour.

Kline, R. (2014) *Putting Patients First. The Duty of Care: Practical Guidance for Healthcare Staff*. Public World, London.
Offers a practical guide that addresses the quality of care provision, safety and professional responsibility.

UNISON (2011) *UNISON Duty of Care Handbook: For Members Working in Health and Social Care*. UNISON, London.
A handbook for health and social care staff that covers care provision, whistle blowing and professional responsibilities.

Chapter 6

Buka, P. (2014) *Patient's Rights, Law and Ethics for Nurses*, 2nd edn. CRC Press, Boca Raton, FL.
Focuses on principles of law and includes clear outlines of the essential legal precedent. Provides a clear understanding not only of basic legal provisions in healthcare, but also of wider issues relating to human rights.

Lee, K. (2015) *A Straightforward Guide to Employment Law: A Comprehensive and Illuminating Guide to all Aspects of Employment Law*. Straight Forward Publishing, Brighton.
A clear and concise guide to all aspects of the law relating to employment rights with changes in the law up to 2015 covered in depth. The book is intended for the layperson but can also be utilised by the professional or the student.

Thompson, N. (2011) *Promoting Equality; Working with Diversity and Difference*, 3rd edn. Palgrave, Basingstoke. Provides those from health and social care backgrounds with a clear guide to the theory and practice of challenging discrimination and promoting equality within the people professions.

Chapter 7

Gates, B. and Mafuba, K. (2015) *Learning Disabilities*. CRC Press, Boca Raton, FL.
The text addresses learning disability nursing from various perspectives, including history and modern-day practice, its role in promoting health and wellbeing, the intersection with mental health, addressing profound disability and people with complex needs, care across the lifespan, forensic settings, and the future of learning disability nursing.
Hewitt-Taylor, J. (2015) *Developing Person Centred Practice. A Practical Approach to Quality Healthcare.* Palgrave, Basingstoke.
A practice-focused exploration of how the idea of person-centredness can be developed and incorporated into everyday health and social care practice.
Kelly, B. (2015) *Dignity, Mental Health and Human Rights, Coercion and the Law*. Ashgate, Farnham.
Explores the human rights consequences of recent and ongoing revisions of mental health legislation. Focuses on dignity, human rights and mental health law to evaluate to what extent the human rights of the mentally ill have been protected and promoted.

Chapter 8

Harvey, N. (2014) *Effective Communication*, 4th edn. Gill & Macmillan, Dublin.
Focuses on the four main communication skills of listening, speaking, reading and writing, incorporating all communications technology. Considers verbal skills, listening skills, and non-verbal and visual communication in one-to-one and group interaction, as well as both personal and work-related settings.
Miller, S. (2015) *Communicating Across Dementia: How to Talk, Listen, Provide Stimulation and Give Comfort*. Robinson, London.
Provides invaluable information for people helping to care for people with dementia at home and also those who do so as part of their job.
Moss, B. (2015) *Communications Skills in Health and Social Care*, 3rd edn. Sage, London.
Presented in a unique, easy-to-use dictionary format, provides a practical guide to help understand and apply the principles of effective communication.
Pavord, E. and Donnelly, E. (2015) *Communication and Interpersonal Skills*, 2nd edn. Lantern Publishing, Banbury.
Offers an introduction to the theory that underpins communication studies and offers opportunities for reflection on practice. Provides helpful guidelines and tips, emphasising that successful communication depends on the quality of the relationship.

Chapter 9

Gates, B., Fearns, D. and Welch, J. (2015) *Learning Disability Nursing at a Glance*. Wiley Blackwell, Oxford.
A user-friendly resource addressing the key principles underpinning contemporary learning disability nursing practice. Relates them to key clinical practice issues, and explores them in the context of maintaining health and wellbeing.
Oliver, D., Foot, C. and Humphries, R. (2014) *Making Our Health and Care Systems Fit for an Ageing Population*. Kings Fund, London.
This text considers how improving services for older people requires us to consider each component of care, as many older people use multiple services.

Pulliam, J. (2011) *The Nursing Assistant. Acute, Subacute and Long Term Care*, 5th edn. Prentice Hall, New Jersey.

A concise, practical and up-to-date guide to the skills today's nursing assistants need to master. The text is North American but nevertheless provides the health and social care worker with principles underpinning care provision.

Chapter 10

Lecko, C. (2013) *Patient Safety and Nutrition and Hydration in the Elderly*. The Health Foundation, London.

Outlines the issues around malnutrition and dehydration that contribute to avoidable harm to people who are cared for or offered support to. Discusses the people most at risk, the most vulnerable: the elderly, those with long-term conditions and the acutely unwell.

Meggitt, C. (2003) *Food Hygiene and Safety: A Handbook for Care Practitioners*. Heinemann, Oxford.

Although dated this text is suitable for those working in social care and early years settings. This handbook covers the issues faced by a range of occupations where people have to handle food.

State of Queensland (Department of Communities, Child Safety and Disability Services) (2012) *Mealtime Support Resources*.

A practical and user-friendly approach to ensure that people enjoy mealtimes and receive appropriate nutritional support. Available at: https://www.communities.qld.gov.au/resources/disability/community-involvement/mealtime-support/mealtime-support-resources.pdf

Chapter 11

Andrews, J. (2015) *Dementia: The One-stop Guide. Practical Advice for Families, Professionals and People Living with Dementia and Alzheimer's Disease*. Profile, London.

A practical guide to dealing with dementia and Alzheimer's.

Barber, C. (2015) *Caring for People with Learning Disabilities: A Guide for Non-Specialist Nurses*. Lantern, Banbury.

This is a concise introduction to the subject covering all aspects of the care and support of the learning disabilities patient, for the non-specialist. Written in a jargon-free style.

Challis, S. (2014) *Understanding Mental Health Problems*. MIND, London.

An introductory booklet to the most common mental health problems, explaining what they are, possible causes and the help available.

Chapter 12

Ash, A. (2014) *Safeguarding Older People from Abuse: Critical Contexts to Policy and Practice*. Policy Press, Bristol.

Focuses on safeguarding older people from abuse. Considers policy and theory with an emphasis on ethics. The text can be rather heavy to read but there are important issues addressed that can help to improve care and support.

Griffiths, R. (2015) Safeguarding vulnerable adults. *British Journal of Nursing* Vol. 24, No. 13, pp. 708–709.

Discusses the professional duty nurses have to safeguard vulnerable adults from abuse. Highlights the fact that all members of the nursing team are well placed to identify and take action to safeguard the vulnerable. Considers how the Care Act 2014 seeks to improve the safeguarding of vulnerable adults.

Office of the Public Guardian (2015) *Safeguarding Policy*. Office of the Public Guardian, Birmingham.

This document produced by the Office of the Public Guardian sets out policy on protecting adults at risk of abuse or neglect.

Chapter 13

McCarthy, T. (2015) *The Common Sense Guide to Improving the Safeguarding of Children: Three Steps to Make a Real Difference*. Jessica Kingsley, London.
Provides purpose and direction in a complex field of work, and offers direct and straightforward guidance on how to improve child protection on the frontline.
Moody, I. (2014) *Nursing and Health Survival Guide: Child Protection: Safeguarding Children Against Abuse*. Routledge, Abingdon.
A pocket-sized guide that will help you develop your understanding of the issues and enable you to identify and respond to difficult child protection concerns with confidence.
Wate, R. (2015) *Multi-agency Safeguarding in a Public Protection World: A Handbook for Protecting Children and Vulnerable Adults*. Pavilion, Brighton.
Addresses adult and child safeguarding issues from a multi-agency perspective. This is a contemporary text with chapters that consider issues such as domestic violence and abuse, internet safeguarding, multi-agency Public Protection Arrangements and safeguarding individuals vulnerable to radicalisation.

255

Chapter 14

Austin, M. (2014) *First Aid Manual: The Authorised Manual of St John Ambulance, St Andrews First Aid and the British Red Cross*, 10th edn. Dorling Kindersley.
A fully authorised first-aid guide endorsed by St John Ambulance, St Andrew's First Aid and the British Red Cross, and packed with step-by-step first aid advice.
Burton, N. (2015) *Clinical Skills for OSCEs*, 5th edn. Scion, Banbury.
Written in a clear and concise way along with easy-to-follow line diagrams and essential clinical photographs. Includes features related to Basic Life Support and Choking.
Resuscitation Council UK (2015) *Immediate Life Support*, 3rd edn. RCUK, London.
Provides healthcare staff with the essential knowledge to treat adult patients in cardiac arrest before the arrival of the resuscitation team or experienced assistance.

Chapter 15

Backcare (2010) *A Carer's Guide to Safer Moving and Handling of People*. Backcare, Teddington.
This text covers important issues such as posture, moving and handling and back care related to those who provide care or offer support to others.
Ludhra, S. (2014) *A Common Sense Guide to Health and Safety at Work*. Routledge, Abingdon.
A short guide for those who need to know more about health and safety in the workplace. Covers all the main aspects of health and safety.
Ruszala, S. (2010) *Moving and Handling People: An Illustrated Guide*. Clinical Skills, London.
An illustrated step-by-step guide to best practice when manual handling of people is needed. Describes principles of safe handling and 24-hour back care in both primary care and secondary care settings.

Chapter 16

Clark, C.L. (2008) *Private and Confidential? Handling Personal Information in the Social and Health Services*. Policy, Bristol.
This book considers key philosophical, ethical and legal issues in the area of privacy and confidentiality, exploring their implications for policy and practice.

Merrix, P. (2012) *Nursing and Health Survival Guide: Record Keeping*. Pearson, Harlow.
Although written for nurses and midwives the principles of record keeping contained in this pocket guide can apply to all settings. It will help you to write clear and concise records.
Thompson, N. (2015) *People Skills*, 4th edn. Palgrave, Basingstoke.
Provides an up-to-date guide on the knowledge and skills required for working successfully with people.

256 Chapter 17

Bissett, L. and Griffith, C. (2014) *The Infection Prevention and Control Handbook*, 2nd edn. Highfield, Doncaster.
Provides a general overview of infection prevention and control. The principles discussed can be applied to any setting.
Department of Health (2013) *Prevention and Control of Infection in Care Homes: An Information Resource*. DH, London.
This resource provides information on the prevention and control of infection in care homes.
Weston, D. (2013) *Fundamentals of Infection Prevention and Control. Theory and Practice*. Wiley Blackwell, Oxford.
Provides the reader with a firm grasp of the principles of infection control, how they relate to clinical practice and the key issues surrounding the subject.

Index

Note: page numbers in *italics* refer to figures; those in **bold** to tables.

Fundamentals of Care: A Textbook for Health and Social Care Assistants, First Edition. Ian Peate.
© 2017 John Wiley & Sons Ltd. Published 2017 by John Wiley & Sons Ltd.